Essential Surgery

Essential Surgery for Nurses

M. A. Henderson MB, ChB, FRCS(Edin)

Consultant Surgeon, Dumfries and Galloway Royal Infirmary

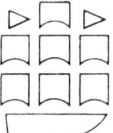

CHURCHILL LIVINGSTONE
EDINBURGH LONDON AND NEW YORK 1980

CHURCHILL LIVINGSTONE
Medical Division of the Longman Group Limited

Distributed in the United States of America by
Churchill Livingstone Inc., 19 West 44th Street, New York,
N.Y. 10036, and by associated companies,
branches and representatives throughout
the world.

© Longman Group Limited 1980

All rights reserved. No part of this publication
may be reproduced, stored in a retrieval system,
or transmitted in any form or by any means,
electronic, mechanical, photocopying, recording
or otherwise, without the prior permission of the
publishers (Churchill Livingstone, Robert Stevenson
House, 1–3 Baxter's Place, Leith Walk,
Edinburgh, EH1 3AF).

First published in 1980
  Reprinted 1980

ISBN 0 443 01737 9

British Library Cataloguing in Publication Data
Henderson, M A
  Essential Surgery for Nurses.
  1. Surgery
  I. Title
  617'.002'4613   RT65   79–41064

Printed in Singapore by Singapore Offset Printing Pte Ltd

Preface

'Not that the story need be long, but it will take a long while to make it short.'
                                                             Henry David Thoreau

My twofold purpose in writing this book was to produce a synopsis of surgery which, firstly, would be of use to nurses in training as an adjunct to a major text book and, secondly, would serve as an aide memoire to nurses and other health care groups, for it covers a wide variety of common surgical conditions.

Much of the text consists of brief summaries, both for ease of learning and reference. However, with many of the conditions, I have devoted text to explaining how the clinical features are caused and why a particular treatment is used. To assist in this, I have included in many of the Chapters brief anatomical and physiological descriptions.

As many diseases have common features and since space is limited, only one explanation is given in the text. The reader is, therefore, asked to bear with the many page references. I hope this will not prove too irritating.

I am greatly indebted to all my nursing and medical friends, who have given much helpful advice and criticism, and who have spent many long hours reading the manuscript.

In this context my special thanks go to Miss A. C. Kelly, Director of Nurse Education, and to Mr D. Shankland, Nurse Tutor, both of South West Scotland College of Nursing, Dumfries.

I have been extremely fortunate in obtaining the services of artist Mrs M. McGee, who produced diagrams of exceptional clarity. My grateful thanks is also offered to Mrs S. Roy for her unstinting secretarial help.

Dumfries, 1979   M.A.H.

Contents

1. Injuries — 1
2. Sinus and fistula — 4
3. Ulcers — 6
4. Infection — 9
5. Lymphatics — 15
6. Tumours — 17
7. Burns — 20
8. Shock — 25
9. Intravenous fluids and electrolytes — 29
10. Blood — 32
11. Blood and vascular disorders — 34
12. Skin — 45
13. Plastic surgery — 48
14. Head and neck — 51
15. Thyroid gland — 58
16. Pharynx — 62
17. Breast — 73
18. Thorax — 77
19. Oesophagus — 87
20. Peritoneum — 93
21. Hernia — 98
22. Stomach and duodenum — 102
23. Intestines — 111
24. Colon and rectum — 120
25. Liver — 131
26. Pancreas — 135
27. Biliary system — 138

28. Brain	142
29. The spine and spinal cord	151
30. Diseases of bone	158
31. Fractures	163
32. Joints	171
33. Dislocation	174
34. Muscles, tendons and bursae	176
35. Kidney	181
36. Bladder	191
37. Prostate and urethra	197
38. Testes	204
Index	209

1 Injuries

Injuries or wounds (i.e. tissue damage) have many causes. The commonest are:
1. Trauma
   a. Sharp as is the incision by a knife.
   b. Blunt as is the blow from a club.
2. Burns
3. Infection

Wounds can be:
1. Closed where the surface, e.g. skin, is intact.
2. Open where the surface, e.g. skin, has been broken.

Closed wounds

These are caused by blunt trauma.

HAEMATOMA

Blood from a burst blood vessel is prevented from spreading by the surrounding tissues and so a collection forms. It can be very small, e.g. subungual haematoma (under the nail; p. 179) or it can be very large, e.g. loin haematoma from a ruptured kidney which may contain several pints of blood (p. 182).

Treatment

Most haematomas are left alone, for usually the blood is reabsorbed within two weeks.

Very large ones are best drained. Others may require draining if they are painful, or if they become infected.

CONTUSION

The tissues are damaged and the blood escapes through the tissue layers. Clinically, the tissues are swollen and tender. If the contusion is superficial, a bruise (echymosis) is seen.

Treatment

Simply rest the affected part. The contusion may be part of more extensive injuries, e.g. following motor accidents.

Open wounds

INCISED WOUNDS

These are due to an injury by a sharp instrument such as a surgeon's

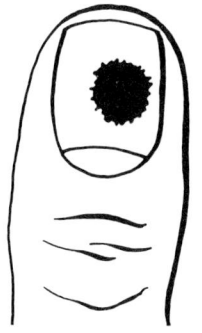

Figure 1.1
Injuries – subungual haematoma

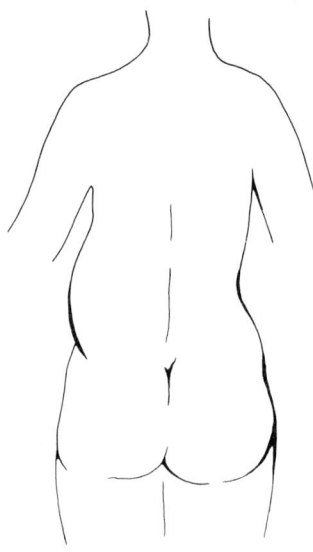

Figure 1.2
Injuries – loin swelling (ruptured kidney)

knife. The clean cut causes minimal trauma. Such wounds heal quickly and well, with a neat scar.

Treatment
1. The wound is cleaned and, if necessary, explored for foreign bodies such as glass.
2. It is then closed by sutures or tape if small.

LACERATED WOUNDS
These wounds have a ragged edge of damaged tissues. They are caused by blunt trauma, e.g. a blow with a club. The tissues burst open with the impact.

Treatment
1. The wound is cleaned.
2. ALL damaged and dead tissues are excised, especially the ragged edges turning the wound as much as possible into an incised wound.
3. The wound is closed with sutures.
4. If there is a great loss of tissues, it may not be possible to close the wound. It is then *treated as a non-specific ulcer* (p. 7), i.e. covered with a dressing and allowed to heal by granulation. Later, if necessary, it is skin grafted.

PENETRATING WOUNDS
These wounds go deeply into the tissues often with only a small skin incision, e.g. knife wounds. Vital organs may be involved and so they must always be treated *seriously*.

Treatment
1. The wound should always be carefully explored. If there is any doubt that it has entered the abdomen, this too must be surgically explored by laparotomy (exploratory operation).

PERFORATING WOUNDS
A wound where the weapon goes completely through the tissues. There is an *entry* and *exit* wound. If caused by a bullet the entry wound is small and the exit wound is large, due to bursting out of the bullet. The damage inside may be greater than is at first supposed, as the bullet may travel 'all over the place', not simply in a straight line between the entry and exit wounds.

Treatment
Perforating wounds require surgical exploration.

N.B. ALL patients who present with open wounds receive Tetanus toxoid to protect them from tetanus (p. 13). Many also receive an antibiotic if the wound is likely to become infected.

Healing of wounds

As with infection, there is local inflammation (p. 9) caused by the chemicals released by the damaged tissues.
1. Initially, the blood clots and forms a clean, efficient dressing.
2. The released chemicals attract white blood cells into the area to remove the dead tissues and any foreign matter.
3. New capillaries are stimulated to sprout from the nearby blood vessels and grow into the clot which is now being digested by the white cells.
4. With the new capillaries there are cells called fibroblasts. They form fibrous tissue, which will become the *scar tissue*.
5. At this stage the mixture of cells and new capillaries is bright red and is called *granulation tissue*.
6. When the granulation tissue reaches the surface the epithelial cells at the edges grow across and so cover it.
7. The newly healed wound is at first red, but the fibrous tissue contracts destroying the capillaries, which are no longer required.

After some months the wound becomes pale. If the granulation tissue grows too quickly for the epithelial cells, it projects above the surface and is called *proud flesh*. This excess will require either to be cut back with a knife or cauterised (destroyed by heat or chemicals e.g. copper sulphate) to allow the epithelial cells to grow over. Sometimes the granulation tissues continue to grow, despite being covered with skin. The scar becomes raised above the surface and is called a *keloid*. It is an over-reaction of healing and may be hereditary. African tribes use it to mark their faces.

Treatment of keloid

Treatment is not to excise, for this makes it worse, but to use steroids applied locally, which dampens down the reaction.

2 Sinus and fistula

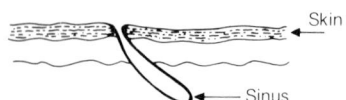

Figure 2.1 Sinus

Sinuses and fistulae are tracks (i.e. tunnels) which run through the tissues.

A sinus is a track from a surface which ends blindly.

A fistula is a track joining two surfaces together.

Aetiology

CONGENITAL
A few are congenital as a result of failure of development, e.g. tracho-oesophageal fistula (p. 88).

ACQUIRED

Acute
Many are formed by an abscess discharging. Discharge to one surface creates a sinus, to two surfaces results in a fistula.

Treatment
They quickly heal if the abscess has drained adequately. Surgical assistance may be required to ensure complete drainage.

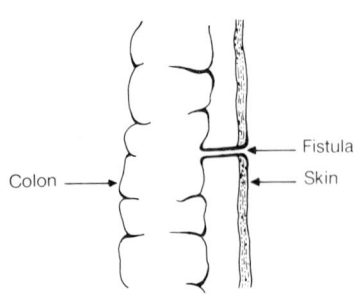

Figure 2.2 Fistula

Chronic
Some persist for various reasons, for example:
1. There is a foreign body present continuing the inflammation.
2. Epithelial cells have grown down the tract converting it to skin (e.g. in ear-piercing).
3. Specific diseases have caused it, e.g. tuberculosis, Crohn's disease (p. 111).
4. Persists because of associated malignant disease.

Treatment
1. Surgical excision of the track and the cause.
2. Special treatment may be needed for the cause, e.g. anti-tuberculous drugs.

Pilonidal sinus

The majority are situated in the natal cleft over the sacrum, where it is seen as a tiny hole with perhaps hair sticking out (pilonidal = hair nest).

Aetiology

It is believed that body hairs work their way or are pushed or squeezed by the buttocks into the skin. The irritation they cause creates the sinus. The sinus may be short and superficial, or it may go deeply into the tissues.

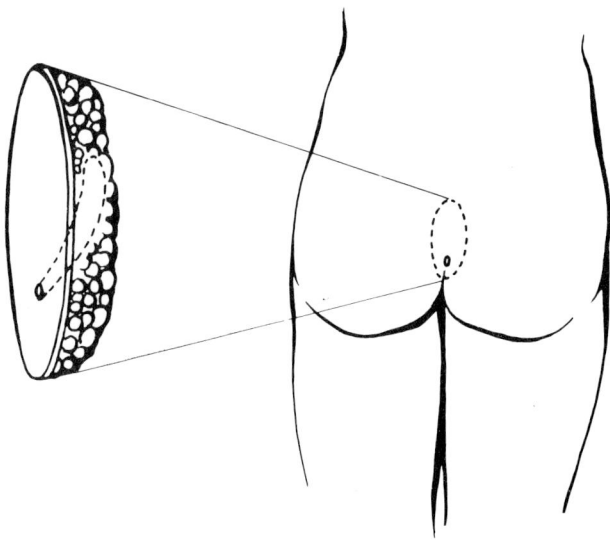

Figure 2.3 Pilonidal sinus

Treatment

To ensure total removal a generous portion of skin and deep tissue round the sinus is excised down to the sacrum. The fairly loose tissues in this region are easily pulled together by sutures closing the gap.

Pilonidal abscess

The entry hole is tiny and easily blocked. Infection can then develop deep to it and an abscess forms. It presents as a tender fluctuant swelling over the sacrum.

Treatment

The abscess is drained and when the inflammation has settled the sinus is excised.

3 Ulcers

An ulcer is a break in the continuity of *any* body surface associated with inflammation. It may be external or internal: an ulcer of the skin or of the intestinal mucosa, e.g. duodenal ulcer.

Description

An ulcer is described by the parts which form it.
1. *The floor* is the centre of the ulcer.
2. *The base* consists of the tissues deep to the floor and surrounding the ulcer.
3. *The edge* is the broken surface running down to the floor.
4. *The discharge* may vary considerably. It may be frank pus, haemorrhagic or clear yellow (serous) fluid.

Stages

Most ulcers go through three stages:
1. *Active extension.* The floor is covered with pus or slough (dead tissue). There is acute inflammation of the edges and the base.
2. *Transitional stage.* The floor is now clean and smooth. The inflammation has settled from the edges and base. There is no obvious healing yet.

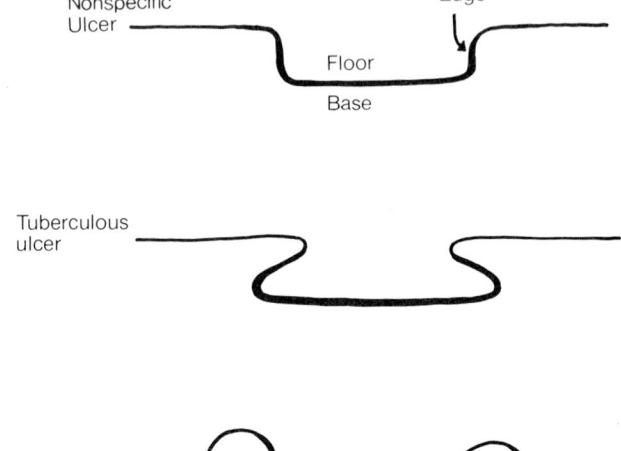

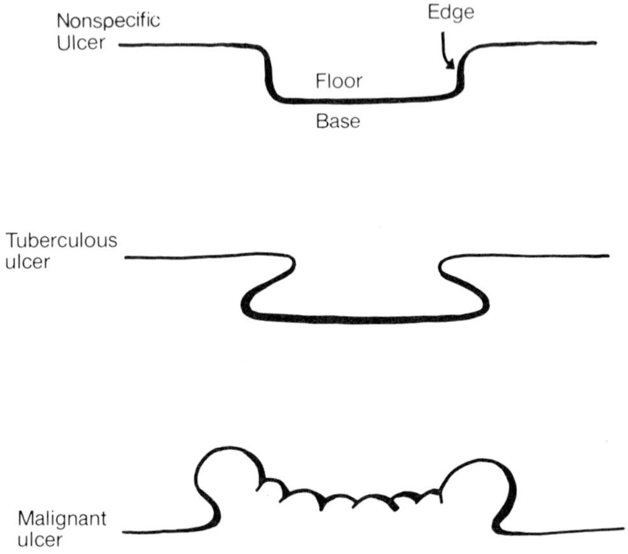

Figure 3.1
Ulcers

3. *Repair stage (healing).* An ulcer heals exactly as any other wound. The base becomes rough with developing granulation tissue. As the granulation tissue reaches the surface the epithelium at the edge are stimulated to divide and grow over the surface. This can be seen as a thin bluish line.

Classification

Ulcers are classified as:
1. Non-specific.
2. Specific.
3. Malignant.

1. NON-SPECIFIC ULCERS
The majority fall into this category, and they have a large variety of causes the commonest being infection and trauma. But a predisposing factor in some is a *poor blood supply* resulting in anoxia and nutritional impairment of the tissues, e.g.

A. Pressure sore
Localised pressure can diminish, or even stop the blood supply to the skin and superficial tissues. This is especially so where they cover, and can be squeezed against underlying bone.

The resultant *anoxic* tissues are thus *much* more liable to ulceration if they are traumatised or become infected. The sacral region and heels are particularly at risk in the bed ridden, but all immobile patients are vulnerable, where their weight is borne for prolonged periods on relatively small areas.

Prevention
a. Frequent changes of position result in much less use of each area and allows recovery of the squeezed tissues.
b. Careful attention is paid to the skin to protect it from trauma and infection.

B. Plaster sore
A particular type of pressure sore caused by an ill fitting plaster cast or splint (p. 165).

C. Varicose ulcer
The inefficient venous drainage causes *anoxia* in the lower limb and predisposes to ulceration (p. 43).

Treatment of non-specific ulcers
a. If possible the cause, if still present, must be removed.
b. The ulcer is kept clean and covered with sterile dressings.
c. If small, it is allowed to heal by granulation. If large, it may require skin grafting.

2. SPECIFIC ULCERS
These ulcers are caused by a specific disease, e.g. tuberculosis, syphilis. They often have special characteristics.

Tuberculous ulcer
This is rare now. The edges are undermined and there is a very scanty discharge.

Treatment of specific ulcers
a. Tuberculous ulcers do not heal until the specific disease causing them is treated, e.g. by antituberculous drugs.
b. They are then treated in the same manners as non-specific ulcers.

3. MALIGNANT ULCERS
These can develop in any malignancy which has developed on a surface, e.g. skin, tongue, stomach. There is a characteristically heaped or rolled edge. The floor is often higher than the surrounding tissue and often indurated. They extend until treated.

Treatment of malignant ulcers
Treatment depends on the site and the type of malignancy (p. 18).

4 Infection

An infection is the invasion of the body by harmful micro organisms. These may be:
1. *Bacteria*, e.g. staphylococcus, causing abscesses.
2. *Viruses*, e.g. mumps, causing parotitis.
3. *Fungi*, e.g. Candida albicans, causing thrush.
4. *Animal parasites*
    a. Protozoa (Unicellular)—Malaria, Amoebic (Dysentery)
    b. Multicellular—worms.

Factors favouring the infection

1. Large numbers of invading organisms.
2. Organisms of a high virulence.
3. Injury to the intact skin or mucous membrane allows entrance to the organisms.
4. Infection of these wounds is greatly increased by the presence of *dead* and *damaged tissues* and *foreign material*, e.g. earth, cloth.
5. Weakened body defences due to *poor diet*, *age* and *illness*, e.g. diabetes.

Body defences against infection

The body reacts at the site of infection with a *local response* (Inflammation) and in severe infections, with a *general systemic response*.

LOCAL RESPONSE—INFLAMMATION
This is the reaction of the local tissues to chemicals released from the damaged tissues, resulting in:
1. *Redness*. The local blood vessels dilate and so bring more blood to the site.
2. *Swelling*. From the dilated vessels—serum pours into the tissues causing a local swelling and bringing white blood cells and antibodies to attack the organisms. It also deposits fibrin at the periphery of the infection, which hinders the spread of the organisms.
3. *Pain*. Due to the swelling, the local nerves become stretched and are stimulated. They are also irritated by the bacterial toxins.
4. *Heat*. The increased blood flow brings more heat to the part affected.

GENERAL SYSTEMIC RESPONSE
1. *Pyrexia*. The body often responds with a high body temperature. This is a defence because many organisms can multiply only at normal body temperature.
2. *Rapid pulse (tachycardia)*. This is caused by the poisons (toxins) from the bacteria acting on the heart and also the result of the increased metabolism, associated with the infection.
3. *Sweating* is a result of the high temperature and high metabolism.
4. *Leucocytosis*. Large numbers of white blood cells, especially polymorphonuclear leucocytes appear in the blood.

Results of infection

Possible results include the following:
1. The infection is destroyed and the part returns to normal.
2. The infection is initially successful and then overcome. Dead body tissues, dead bacteria and leucocytes which may then form an abscess.
3. The infection may spread locally resulting in a cellulitis.
4. The infection may overwhelm the defences spreading through the blood resulting in bacteraemia (p. 11), septicaemia (p. 11) or pyaemia (p. 11).

Local complications of infection

CELLULITIS
This is a spreading of the organism through the tissues, usually associated with streptococcal infections (p. 12) and it is often very rapid and may be fatal.

Clinical features
The clinical features are those of red swollen painful tissues, associated with general signs of infection.

Treatment
1. Rest and elevation of the part.
2. Incision if pus is thought to be present.
3. Antibiotics, e.g. benzyl penicillin 2 to 4 g/day (Streptococci are very sensitive to it).

ABSCESS
This is the result of the infection becoming localised. As the volume of pus increases it tends to follow the line of least resistance (tracking) i.e. to the skin, or to the bowel where it discharges (pointing).

Clinical features
1. There is a localised red fluctuant swelling, which is warm to the touch and very tender.

2. When pointing the skin becomes increasingly shiny and red, and the pus appears as a yellow centre.
3. There may be a general systemic response if the abscess is large.

Treatment
1. Incision and drainage.
2. Antibiotics—decided by the culture and the sensitivity of the bacteria.

LYMPHANGITIS
Inflammation of the lymphatic channels leading to the draining lymph glands. Nearly always the result of *streptococcal infection*. Presents as tender red lines running to the lymph glands from the site of infection.

Treatment
Antibiotics (Benzyl penicillin) for the primary infection.

LYMPHADENITIS
Frequently in infection the draining lymph glands become inflamed and enlarged (p. 26).

General complications of infection

BACTERAEMIA
Bacteraemia means bacteria in the blood and may not be particularly significant. Bacteria are usually dealt with very quickly by the defence mechanisms, but occasionally they may infect damaged or weakened areas.

SEPTICAEMIA
This is bacteria in very large numbers in the blood and is very serious. The bacteria may even multiply in the blood.

Clinical features
1. A very high peaking temperature and pulse.
2. A shivering attack (rigor).
3. A return to normal with sweating.
4. Leucocytosis.

The bacteria are dealt with by the defences, but they have a better chance to settle out and can cause abscesses in organs throughout the body.

PYAEMIA
Small collections of organisms matted together with blood clot circulating in the blood (infected emboli) (p. 36). This is very serious and may cause multiple abscesses.

Bacteria

Commensals
Harmless bacteria which live on the body surfaces. Some commensals when given the right condition become pathogens, e.g. *E. coli.* and *staphylococcus aureus.*

Pathogens
Harmful bacteria. They may be harmful either by their direct local action or by poisons (toxins) they release, which have general systemic effects (*C. tetani*).

Common infections

STAPHYLOCOCCUS AUREUS
This is normally a commensal in the nose and in body folds, e.g. axilla.

Causes
Boils, breast abscesses, hospital wound infections, bacteraemia and septicaemia.

STREPTOCOCCUS PYOGENES
May also be carried in the nose.

Causes
Tonsillitis, sinusitis, puerperal fever. It also produces a toxin called 'the spreading factor' which allows it to spread quickly through the tissues. This causes a widespread inflammation (cellulitis, p. 10) called *erysipelas.*

COLIFORM BACILLI
There are many different types. Most are in the large bowel as commensals. They become pathogenic in certain conditions.

Causes
Urinary infections, wound infections, bacteraemia and septicaemia. They are a common cause of bacteraemic shock (p. 26).

Less common infections

CLOSTRIDIUM TETANI
This is a normal commensal of the large bowel of cattle. It passes in their faeces into the farm land where it can survive a very long time. Where soil contaminates wounds, there is a danger of it becoming a pathogen.

Clinical features
The bacteria produce a toxin which, becoming attached to nerves, causes muscle spasm. The face muscles are the first affected (lockjaw).

The quicker the onset of symptoms after the injury the more severe they are.

Mild cases may only have facial spasm (Risus sardonicus—sardonic smile).

Severe cases have all muscles affected and the muscle spasm may stop respiration and cause death.

Treatment

The following treatment has largely superseded the previously used horse antitoxin serum (ATS) which can cause severe anaphylactic reactions (p. 26).
1. Penicillin in large doses is given to kill the bacteria, 1 million units four-hourly.
2. The wound is opened and meticulously cleaned.
3. In mild cases, sedatives are used to relax the muscle spasm.
4. In severe cases, the muscles are paralysed with a relaxant (e.g. tubocurarine). The patient's respiration is maintained through a tracheostomy by positive pressure respiration (p. 80). Recovery may take weeks.

Prevention

Young children are now given an altered toxin (toxoid) routinely and this stimulates immunity. Everyone can be protected in this way. However, the immunity gradually wanes and requires reinforcing after some years. *All* patients with wounds receive toxoid either to initiate their immunity or to boost their previously acquired immunity (0.5 ml Tetanus toxoid subcutaneously). Antitetanus toxoid (ATT) does not cause anaphylaxis.

GAS GANGRENE

This is a clinical condition which occurs with simultaneous infection by several organisms. The main one is *Clostridium welchii*. This bacteria and the others are normally commensals in the bowel of animals and man.

Clinical features
1. The bacteria attack body tissues, especially muscle and in doing so produce a foul smelling gas.
2. The wound may bubble and the gas in the tissues crackles on palpation (crepitation).
3. The patient becomes very seriously ill and may die from the bacterial toxins released into the circulation.

Treatment
1. Adequate removal of all infected tissues.
2. Washing the tissues with hydrogen peroxide (the bacteria are very sensitive to oxygen).
3. Anti gas gangrene serum and antibiotics.
4. It may be necessary to amputate a limb to remove the source of the toxins.

Prevention
It is important that wounds, especially those involving muscles are adequately cleansed and all damaged tissues, especially muscle, are removed.

Chronic infections

TUBERCULOSIS
No longer common in developed countries, but very common still in the Third World. There are two main types of bacillus:
1. Human type.
2. Bovine type (in cattle).

Both infect humans. The *human* type affects mainly the lungs, from droplet infections from others, e.g. coughing. The *bovine* type, from infected milk, often affects the small bowel.

The infection usually causes a chronic inflammation, which may go on to abscess formation (p. 10). It often spreads to the local lymph glands which become enlarged and may break down and form abscesses. The infection can spread by the blood to infect any organ or part of the body, causing, for example

Tuberculous meningitis.
Tuberculous osteomyelitis and arthritis.
Tuberculous kidneys and bladder.

Clinical features
1. The patient feels unwell.
2. There is often a night time pyrexia and night sweats.
3. Local signs develop of the infection, e.g. cough.

Any tuberculous abscess forms slowly and presents as a soft fluctuant swelling, which is only slightly tender and red. It is therefore called a *cold abscess* (because of the lack of acute symptoms).

Treatment

Medical
This is usually all that is required using anti-tuberculous drugs, often in combination, such as *rifampicin* (450 to 600 mg/day), *ethambutol* (1 g/day) and *isoniazid* (500 mg/day).

Surgery
1. May be required to drain a cold abscess.
2. To remove a badly infected or destroyed organ, e.g. kidney.

5 Lymphatics

Lymphadenopathy

Diseases of the lymph glands.

AETIOLOGY
1. Infection—bacterial or viral—lymphadenitis.
2. Malignant
   a. Primary (see below)
   b. Secondary (metastatic spread).

Lymphadenitis

Inflammation of the lymph glands can be *acute* or *chronic* and has many causes.

ACUTE
1. Direct—viral infection.
2. Indirect—infection may be carried to them by the lymphatics.

Clinical features
1. The lymph glands enlarge and are tender to palpation.
2. They may become the site of abscess formation if the infection is very severe.
3. Whole groups of glands may be enlarged by viral infections, e.g. cervical glands in glandular fever, mesenteric glands in mesenteric adenitis (p. 114).

Treatment
The treatment varies greatly, depending on the cause.

CHRONIC
This is the result of a chronic infection such as tuberculosis or continuing infection, e.g. from carious teeth (cervical glands).

Clinical features
1. The glands are enlarged but less tender.
2. An abscess is less likely except in tuberculosis.

Treatment
The treatment varies, depending on the cause.

Primary malignant disease

There are several different types of malignant disease which arise in the lymphoid tissue—*lymphoma, lympho sarcoma, lymphadenoma (Hodgkins disease)*.

As a group they are called the *reticuloses.*

Clinical features
1. One or more lymph glands become enlarged, and are painless.
2. There may be a general systemic upset with malaise, anaemia, pyrexia.

Treatment
1. A biopsy is taken of the enlarged gland to confirm the diagnosis.
2. Lymphangiograms may be carried out to determine the extent of the disease (see below).
3. Radiotherapy or cytotoxics are the usual method of treatment.

Secondary malignant disease

Malignant tumours, especially carcinomas, invade the lymphatics and are carried to the lymph glands (p. 18).

Lymphangiogram

Radio-opaque dye is injected into a lymphatic channel in the foot or hand. The dye travels with the lymph to the lymph glands. These can be outlined by X-ray examination and involvement in disease demonstrated.

6 Tumours

Tumours are new cell growths (neoplasm) where the dividing of the cells (mitosis) is not controlled by the body and serves no useful function for the body.

The main differences are as follows:

Benign
1. It has a capsule
2. It does not locally invade
3. It does not travel to distant sites
4. It does not kill

Malignant
1. It has no capsule
2. It invades locally
3. It metastasises (spreads) to distant sites
4. It kills the host

But there are exceptions:
1. Some benign tumours can kill by their sheer size, e.g. ovarian.
2. Some malignant tumours do not metastasise, e.g. rodent ulcer.
3. Some benign tumours can become malignant, e.g. bladder.

Benign tumours

These may arise from most body tissues.
1. *Epithelial or endothelial cells* } Papilloma arise from these, e.g. skin, bladder, (p. 194) colon. They may become malignant.
2. *Skin pigment cells:* naevus (beauty spot).
3. *Glandular*—adenoma: breast (p. 75), parotid (p. 56), thyroid (p. 60).
4. *Blood vessels*—haemangioma: two types.
   a. Capillary: birth mark; port wine stain of skin.
   b. Cavernous: a purple nodule which blanches on pressure.
5. *Fibrous tissue*—fibroma: presents as a nodule. Can arise in most situations.
6. *Fat*—lipoma: a soft swelling, especially common subcutaneously.
7. *Osteoma*
8. *Chondroma* } Simple bone and cartilage tumours (p. 161).
9. *Myoma:* a simple muscle tumour, the commonest site being the uterus—fibroid or fibromyoma.

TREATMENT
Most simple tumours are excised locally for one or more of the following reasons:
1. To establish or confirm the diagnosis.
2. To exclude or prevent malignancy.
3. For cosmetic reasons.

Malignant tumours

1. *Epithelial or endothelial cells.*
   a. Carcinoma: these are named after the original tissue, e.g. squamous carcinoma of skin (p. 46). Transitional cell carcinoma of bladder (p. 194).
   b. Melanoma: malignant tumour of the pigment cells of the skin.
2. *Gland tissue:* Adenocarcinoma, e.g. of the breast (p. 75) or stomach (p. 109).
3. *Connective tissues:* sarcoma—these are much less common. Fibrosarcoma from fibrous tissue, osteogenic sarcoma (p. 162) from bone, myosarcoma from muscle.
4. *Lymph glands.* A variety of malignant disease is found in lymphoid tissue (reticulo endothelial tissue) with varying degrees of malignancy, e.g. lymphoma, reticulo sarcoma, Hodgkin's disease (see p. 16).
5. *Leukaemia.* Malignant disease of parent cells which produce the white blood cells. There are two main types:
   a. Lymphatic leukaemia arises in the lymphoid tissues and
   b. Myeloid leukaemia in the bone marrow. The peripheral blood becomes filled with primitive inactive lymphocytes or polymorpholeucocytes respectively.

Well-differentiated tumours resemble the original parent cells.

Anaplastic tumours have bizarre cells which have lost all likeness to the original cells. Tumours of this type are usually much more malignant.

MODES OF SPREAD
1. *Local.* The tumour cells infiltrate the neighbouring healthy cells. (To be sure all the tumour has been excised, surgeons remove a cuff of surrounding healthy tissue).
2. *Along natural passages*, e.g. detached cells pass in the urine from a tumour in the pelvis of the kidney (p. 188) and may become implanted in the ureter or bladder mucosa (p. 194).
3. *Across serous cavities*, e.g. a tumour of the stomach may penetrate through the peritoneal coat of stomach and detached cells can become implanted in the surface of other organs, so invading it, e.g. ovary.
4. *Lymphatics.* Tumours, especially carcinomas, invade the lymphatics and detached cells pass with the lymph to the lymph glands. The cells multiply and the glands enlarge, being replaced with malignant cells. Eventually, further cells pass on to enter the blood stream via the thoracic duct. Carried in the blood to distant organs, they settle producing secondary tumours (metastases).
5. *Blood spread.* Tumours especially sarcomas can invade blood vessel walls and so enter the blood stream directly.

METHODS OF TREATMENT

1. *Surgery*. The aim is
   a. To remove the tumour by wide excision through surrounding healthy tissues.
   b. To remove all draining lymph glands in case they are involved.
2. *Radiotherapy*. The effect is *to stop the cells dividing* and eventually they die. It may be used alone or in combination with surgery to catch any residual tumour locally or in the lymph glands.
3. *Hormones*. Some carcinomas of the breast are dependent on the oestrogen level in the blood. Lowering the level (by removing the ovaries) may shrink the tumour. This never totally destroys the tumour and so is palliative only. The drug Tamoxifen prevents the hormone from reaching the tumour and has a similar effect (p. 76).

   Carcinoma of the prostate is also hormone-dependent, being stimulated by male hormone (testosterone) and inhibited by oestrogens (p. 199).
4. *Cytotoxics*. These drugs interfere with the metabolism of dividing cells and especially tumour cells. They are used in combination and are very effective against leukaemias. However, they also affect normal cells (especially the marrow) and must be used with extreme caution.

7 Burns

Causes

1. Heat. But burns can also be caused by:
2. Cold.
3. Electricity.
4. Radiation.
5. Chemicals.
6. Ultra-violet light (sun-burn).

The body responds to burns, as to any other injury, by inflammation and then healing.

Classification

1. Superficial.
2. Deep.

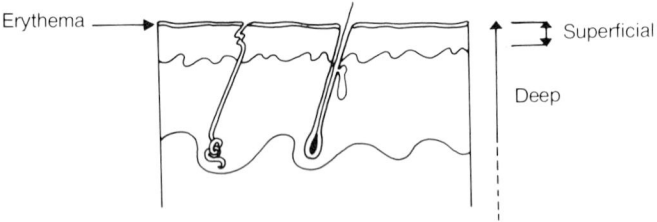

Figure 7.1
Superficial and deep burns

SUPERFICIAL BURN
Where some of the germinal layer of the epithelium survives, in the sweat glands and the hair follicles.

Clinical feature
Blistering is the typical sign of a superficial burn.

There is an outpouring of fluid from the deeper injured layers, which lifts the superficial, burnt (dead) surface.

The blisters often burst leaving a red raw surface, which oozes serous fluid, and may bleed.

Superficial burns are painful, for nerve endings are exposed and inflamed.

Healing
The deeper cells which have survived start to divide and cover the raw surface. There is little or no scarring.

Erythema
There is much less heat and no blistering, but enough to cause slight injury and so inflammation causing vasodilatation, leading to redness, a feeling of heat, tenderness and oedema, e.g. mild sun-burn.

DEEP BURN
In this type of burn the heat is greater, or applied for longer. All the epithelial elements of the skin are destroyed. It can be said the skin is 'cooked', i.e. the protein is coagulated (as the white of an egg is cooked). In extreme cases, the burn can be very deep, involving muscle and even bone.

Clinical features
1. The skin, at first glance, may look nearly normal.
2. Then it is noticed that it is shiny and the blood vessels are easily seen.
3. But the blood in them cannot be squeezed out, as it has been coagulated.
4. The skin is very firm to the touch (like leather).
5. It is uncomfortable, but not painful for most of the nerve endings are also dead.
6. There will be no bleeding from any cut.
7. Sometimes there is charring and blackening.

This dead surface tissue is called the *eschar*.

Healing
In the depths where the tissues have survived the injury stimulates granulation tissue (p. 3) which grows and separates the dead eschar creating in effect a large ulcer (p. 6). As all the epithelial elements are dead, skin cover must grow in from the edges, which takes a very long time.

Meanwhile the granulation tissue continues to form fibrous tissue, which becomes scar tissue. When healing is complete there is large amounts of scar tissue, which contracts (p. 3) causing great distortion of the surface and limitation of joint movement. This is one reason why the surgeon is so anxious to get the surface healed with grafts as quickly as possible.

Assessment of burns

This is vital to the treatment of the patient.

THE RULE OF NINES
The body surface is divided into percentages so that an arm is 9 per cent, and the front of the trunk is 18 per cent. The total percentage of the body surface burnt is measured by simple addition.

It is important also to calculate how much of the burn is superficial and how much is deep, despite the difficulty in being accurate on occasions.

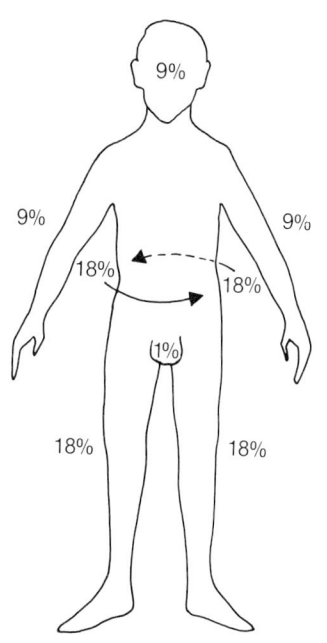

Figure 7.2
Burns – percentage areas – rule of nine

Thus, a burn of the chest (half front of trunk) and two arms is 27 per cent, of which one-third of the total could be superficial, and two-thirds could be deep.

Treatment of burns

The treatment is divided into:
1. Resuscitation of the patient.
2. Local treatment of the burns.

RESUSCITATION
This takes absolute priority over the local treatment (burns meanwhile are covered with sterile towels).

Respiration
Respiration may be in danger from oedema if the burn is around the mouth or pharynx, and the patient may require an immediate tracheostomy.

Shock
Shock is often present in severe burns (10 per cent or more), and can be profound and severe. It is caused by:
1. Fluid loss.
2. Toxins.
3. Pain.

Fluid loss
Superficial burns lose fluid from:
1. Blisters.
2. Oozing.
3. Oedema (oedema fluid is 'out of circulation' and not useful).

Deep burns lose fluid mainly from oedema.
The fluid loss if either type of burn is over 15 per cent (10 per cent in children) must be replaced immediately by intravenous fluids. The amount needed is calculated by formulae based on the percentage of burn and the weight of the patient:

Percentage of burn $\times$ kg patient's weight $\times 2 =$ Total fluid lost by burn in ml in the first 24 hours.

Example:
An 18 per cent burn in a 70 kg man

$18 \times 70 \times 2 = 2520$ ml

Treatment for shock:
In superficial burns 50 per cent or more is given as dextran or plasma, the rest mainly as $\bar{N}$ saline.
In deep burns, where blood is destroyed, whole blood is given instead of dextran or plasma.
In addition to the burns-replacement fluid the patient's daily require-

ment of 2 200 ml must also be given (p. 29).
Therefore *total adult fluid* required is

2 520 ml replacement + 2 200 requirement = 4 720 ml/24 hours.

These are rough forecasts and are modified as necessary by:
1. Monitoring the replacement by a CVP line (p. 27).
2. Maintaining an adequate urinary output—0·75 ml/kg/hour.
3. Frequent electrolyte and haemoglobin checks.

Toxins
These come from the burnt tissue. It is most important to reduce their effect by dilution with adequate intravenous fluids and to promote their excretion by maintaining a good urinary output.

Pain
Analgesics are given and this helps to combat the shock.

Catheterisation
Catheterisation may be necessary where there is burning of the genitalia and is also of great assistance in assessing the hourly urine output.

Tetanus toxoid
Tetanus toxoid is given routinely as for any wound.

Antibiotics
Systemic antibiotics are given in severe burns, e.g. ampicillin 2 g/day.

LOCAL TREATMENT OF BURNS

First objective
To get healing as quickly as possible, so there will be the least amount of fibrous tissue formed, thus minimising the scarring and contractures.

Second objective
To prevent *infection* which is the greatest hindrance to rapid healing. Therefore all but patients with minor burns should be nursed in single cubicles.

Methods
1. Open (exposure) method.
2. Closed (dressings) method.

Open method
Designed to create dry, cool conditions hostile to bacteria.
1. The burns are cleaned with mild antiseptic (Savlon 1:80) and all blisters are opened. All loose tissue is excised.
2. The raw surface oozing serum is exposed. The serum gradually dries to a crust, which is a perfect dressing for the healing taking place beneath.

A deep burn is similarly treated, for the dead tissue sterilised by the heat is also a perfect dressing.
3. After 14 to 21 days the granulation tissue starts to separate either the crust or the dead tissue. Infection can now get beneath them. To stop this, the crust or dead tissue must be removed.
4. If it was a superficial burn, it will now be healed, or nearly so.
5. If deep, the raw area is skin grafted or covered with dressings until it can be skin grafted. (This is now the closed method).

Closed method

Used where it is not possible to expose, e.g. the patient has to rest on part of the trunk.
1. The burns are cleaned and treated as for the exposure methods, with blisters opened and loose tissue excised.
2. Antibiotic powder is applied and the burn covered with sterile non-stick dressings. With superficial burns, there is much oozing (see open method) and the dressings require considerable padding.
3. The dressings are changed every three to four days.
4. At two to three weeks the burnt surface will be healing and separating the dead tissue. This is therefore removed. Superficial burns will be healed. Deep burns will require grafting or covered with dressings until they can be grafted.

GENERAL CONSIDERATION
1. Patients with burns require a high protein diet for healing.
2. A careful watch is kept to make sure they do not become anaemic.
3. Any sign of infection (such as pyrexia) requires a change of dressings and possibly systemic antibiotics.
4. Where the patient cannot supply enough for his own skin for grafting it is possible to use skin from someone else (homograft) (p. 50). This will take for a time, but will be rejected. It does, however, give a good cover temporarily.

Similarly porcine (pig) skin suitably prepared is used. It does not 'take', but gives a very close cover. It requires frequent renewal.

8 Shock

Shock is a sudden fall in the blood pressure, severe enough to endanger life. Blood pressure is the pressure created by the heart pushing the blood through the blood vessels.

Shock can be divided into two main groups, cardiogenic and hypovolaemic.

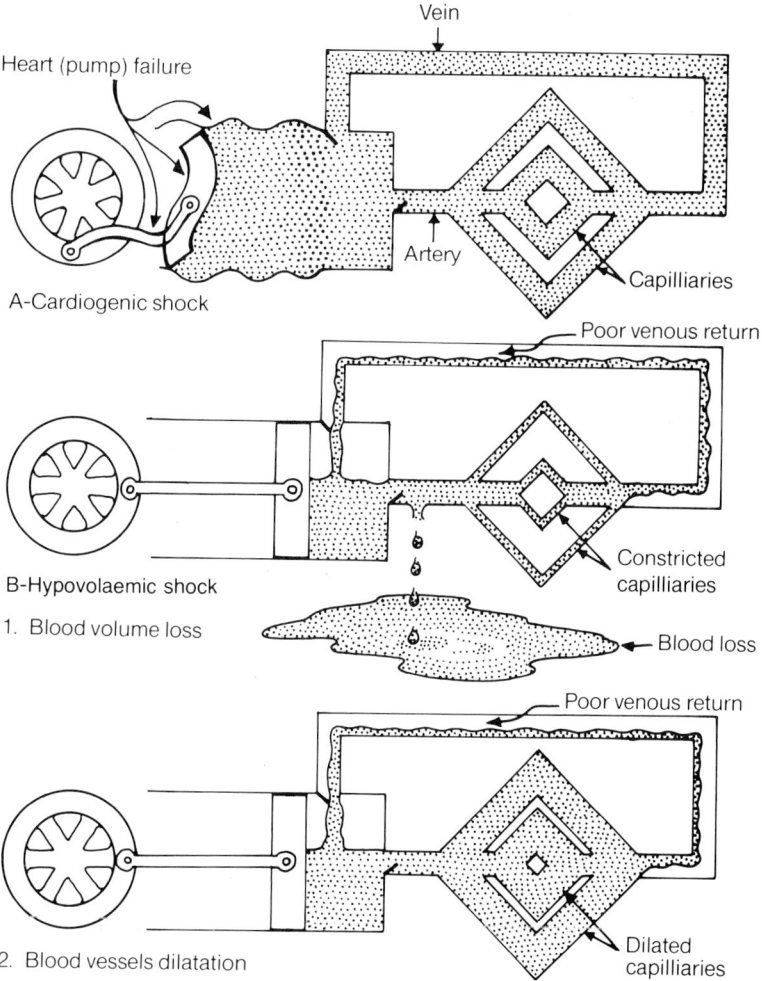

Figure 8.1
Shock

Cardiogenic shock

The heart may fail to maintain its pumping action and the blood pressure will fall. This failure is seen in cases of myocardial infarction where shock is not infrequently present.

Hypovolaemic shock

The result of violent change in either:
1. The blood volume or
2. The capacity of the blood vessels.

THE BLOOD VOLUME
In severe fluid loss there is not enough blood to fill the vessels and the pressure falls, e.g. following haemorrhage—haemorrhagic shock.

THE BLOOD VESSELS
The capacity of blood vessels can be altered greatly if they dilate suddenly, so creating much more space for the blood. The blood fills the extra space and much less returns by the vena cavae to the heart. The blood pressure falls as there is now less to be pushed out into the aorta (p. 27).

This dilatation occurs as a result of stimulation of the autonomic nervous system which acts mainly on the small vessels, especially those in the abdominal cavity.

Causes of dilatation

1. Neurogenic or vaso vagal shock
The result of a severe fright or severe pain. The brain stimulates the autonomic nervous system via the *vagus nerve*. It is often very temporary (simple faint) and may require no treatment, or it can be very severe.

2. Anaphylactic shock
The result of an allergic person receiving a dose of the allergen. There may be profound shock, the result of the release of histamine into the circulation dilating the blood vessels, e.g. incompatible blood transfusion (p. 32).

3. Bacteraemic or endotoxic shock
The result of a severe infection, where large amounts of toxins enter the circulation. *E. coli* is a common cause often with a septicaemia (p. 11). It is very serious and carries a high mortality.

Clinical features

1. Rapid weak pulse and low systolic and diastolic blood pressure.
2. Cold sweaty skin and pallor.

3. Restlessness and the patient is very frightened.
4. Deep sighing respiration.
5. No urine is secreted if the pressure falls below about 80 mmHg.

Treatment (see Table 8.1)

Cardiac shock is a medical problem.
All other types of shock, if severe, require:

1. *Intravenous drip* to
a. Replace blood in haemorrhagic shock.
b. Fill up the dilated blood vessels with fluids in non-haemorrhagic shock this can be plasma substitute—dextran (p. 33).

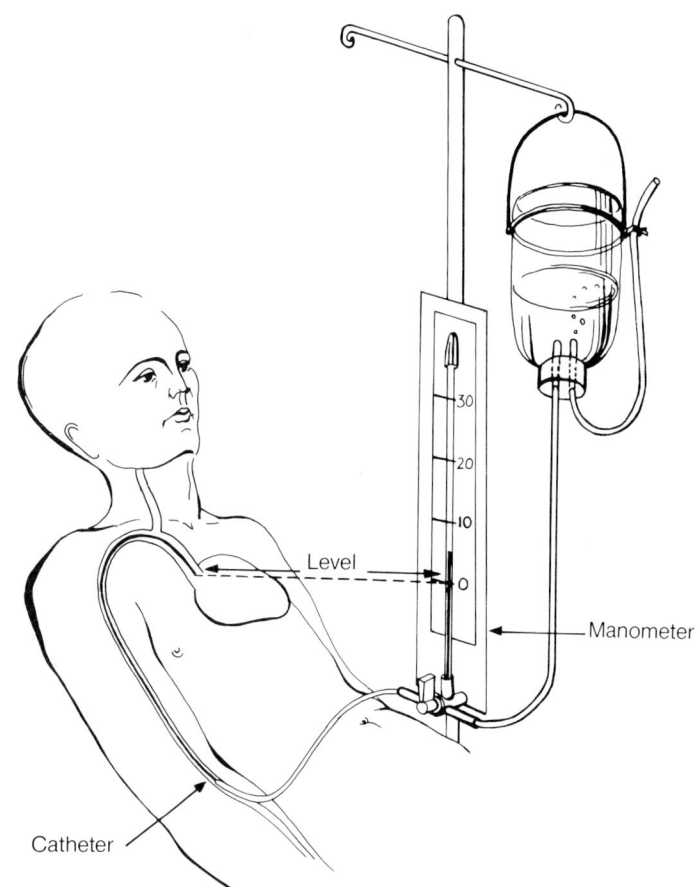

Figure 8.2
Intravenous infusion for measuring central venous pressure

Central venous pressure line (c.v.p.) measures the amount of blood returning to the heart.

A catheter is passed through an arm vein so that the tip lies in the superior vena cava next to the right atrium. The pressure in the cava is measured (c.v.p.). This pressure depends on the venous return or volume which is very low in hypovolaemic shock (p. 26). Fluid is transfused until the pressure returns to normal (5 to 10 cm of water pressure).

2. *Raising the foot of the bed* and draining the blood from the legs into the trunk will give a temporary improvement (500 ml).

3. *Steroids* are used in anaphylactic shock and often in bacteraemic shock.

4. *Antibiotics* are essential in bacteraemic shock.

5. *Oxygen.* This makes sure that the full oxygen carrying capacity of the blood is utilised.

Table 8.1 Treatment of shock

Type of shock	Blood	Plasma or substitute	Oxygen	Steroids	Antibiotics
Haemorrhagic	+		+		
Neurogenic or Vasovagal		+(?)	+(?)		
Anaphylactic		+	+	+	
Bacteraemic		+	+	+	+

9 Intravenous fluids and electrolytes

A patient's *intake* of fluid must equal the *output* of fluid (see Table 9.1).

Table 9.1 Average daily fluid balance

Intake		Output	
From metabolism	500 ml	Lungs	500 ml
With food	500 ml	Skin	500 ml
As liquids	1 200 ml	Faeces	200 ml
		Urine	1 000 ml
Total	2 200 ml		2 200 ml

Note. Both sides of the equation have invisible portions. On the output side (lungs, skin, faeces) this is called the *insensible water loss*.

There may be abnormal fluid losses such as in diarrhoea, vomiting, or from post-operative drains and these must also be recorded.

Electrolyte balance

The different salts in the body, being in solution are split into two parts which are collectively called the electrolytes. They are vital not only for the proper function of the body but also in maintaining the correct acid-base balance of the body—the pH. They are measured in the blood in units called millimoles per litre (mmol/l), and they vary within fairly narrow margins. They can be divided broadly into two groups of acid (negative) and alkaline (positive) electrolytes, and they balance one another—acid-base (alkali) balance (see Table 9.2).

Table 9.2 Normal electrolyte balance

Alkaline		Acid	
Sodium (Na^+)	135–145 mmol/l	Chloride (Cl^-)	95–106 mmol/l
Potassium (K^+)	3.5–4.5 mmol/l	Phosphate (PO_4^{--})	0.8–1.45 mmol/l
Calcium (Ca^+)	2.25–2.5 mmol/l	Bicarbonate (HCO_3^{--})	22–30 mmol/l

As with fluid, the *intake* and *output* must balance:

Output			*Intake*
Sodium Chloride	80 mmol of sodium and chloride/day	equals	5 g of salt or 560 ml of N saline (p. 30)
Potassium	40 mmol/day	equals	3 g of potassium (chloride)

In disease, there may be great losses of electrolytes. For example:
1. Sodium and potassium loss is high with intestinal disease and diarrhoea.
2. Potassium and chloride loss is high in cases of continuous vomiting.

3. In continuous vomiting acid is also lost and the now excess base causes the pH to rise (metabolic alkalosis).
4. Acid-base balance may be altered e.g. toxic diseases and uncontrolled diabetes produce acid. The pH becomes less and the bicarbonate level in the blood falls as it is used to neutralise the acid (metabolic acidosis).

Urea

Urea (2·5 to 7·5 mm/l) is the product of protein metabolism. The blood level may rise from *increased formation* in toxic illnesses, where tissue proteins are being destroyed or following gastro-intestinal haemorrhage where there is *increased absorption* by the gut of breakdown products from the blood.

It is excreted by the kidneys and levels also rise from *impaired excretion* in renal failure and *dehydration* where little urine is formed.

Intravenous fluids

These fluids are used intravenously to replace the loss of fluid and electrolytes when oral fluid intake is not possible. Water alone cannot be used in large quantities intravenously for it causes breakdown (haemolysis) of the red blood corpuscles.

SALINE SOLUTIONS
The commonest is 0·9 per cent saline, which has the same amount of sodium and chloride as plasma. This is called N̄ saline or Normal saline and does not affect the red cells. It not only replaces fluid, but also salt. Other strengths can be used.

DEXTROSE SOLUTIONS (SUGAR)
The commonest is 5 per cent Dextrose, which is compatible with plasma. It supplies calories and fluid. Other strengths can be used.

DEXTROSE-SALINE SOLUTIONS
This is a combination of the above, supplying fluid, calories and salt.

POTASSIUM
The above solutions are now available with potassium; or, it can be added separately as potassium chloride solution.

Table 9.3 Post-operative patient (i.e. short-term replacement)

Requirement/daily	Given/daily
5 g Sodium chloride	500 ml N̄ saline
2000–2500 ml/water	1500–2000 ml dextrose solution

Note
1. Patients may require more fluid and electrolytes if fluid is lost by drain and suction.
2. Potassium is not required in the short term.

BICARBONATE

Sodium bicarbonate solutions are available to correct severe acidosis (p. 30), especially after cardiac arrest.

Intravenous feeding

Where patients are on prolonged intravenous therapy they can receive not only carbohydrate replacement by dextrose, but *amino acids* to replace their normal dietary protein.

Emulsified fats are also available to be given intravenously and they are used by the body as a productive source of calories.

Proprietory sources of these are available:

Amino acids. Aminosol, Aminoplex, Vamin.

Emulsified fat. Intra lipid.

10 Blood

Blood is divided into four Groups A, B, AB and O depending on the antigens A and B, which are in the red cells (O has none). The *plasma* contains the opposite antibody.

i.e. Group A (antigen A) contains antibody B (Anti-B)
　　Group B contains antibody A (Anti-A)
　　Group AB contains *no* antibody.
　　Group O contains anti-A and anti-B.

The red cells may or may not contain another antigen called the *rhesus factor*, but the normal plasma contains *no* antibody against it. But it will develop in Rh −ve patients if they are given Rh +ve cells. They will react at the next transfusion of Rh +ve cells, causing haemolysis (destruction) of the red cells.

It is vital that the *red cells* of one group do not mix with the plasma of an incompatible group for the *red cells* will be attacked and coagulated together. This is an incompatible transfusion and must be stopped immediately.

Clinical features of an incompatible transfusion

1. Rigors with pyrexia.
2. Back pain.
3. Anaphylactic shock.
4. Oliguria—a very small urinary output.

BLOOD TRANSFUSION
To prevent reactions during a transfusion the blood of the donor must be 'matched' with that of the patient.

In an extreme emergency Group O Rh −ve blood can be given to anyone, for the red cells contain *no* ABO antigens (universal donor) and will not be attacked, otherwise ALL blood must be 'MATCHED' to the patient.

PACKED RED CELLS
The red cells can be concentrated by the removal of part of the plasma, so reducing the bulk of the transfusion. It is used where only red cells are required, e.g. severe anaemia.

PLASMA
Where red cells have not been lost, e.g. superficial burns, plasma alone is used to replace fluid lost.

PLASMA SUBSTITUTES
These contain chemical substitutes for the plasma proteins and they can be used instead of plasma, e.g. dextran.

11 Blood and vascular disorders

HAEMORRHAGE
Haemorrhage is the escape of blood from the vascular system. It may be:
1. Arterial—bright red blood is pumped out.
2. Venous—dark red blood flows as a steady stream.
3. Capillary—Seen as a general oozing from a raw surface.

PRIMARY HAEMORRHAGE
Haemorrhage at the time of injury. It is stopped by the blood clotting and by retraction of vessel wall. In severe haemorrhage, the low blood pressure helps these to take place.

REACTIONARY HAEMORRHAGE
New haemorrhage after several hours. The clot is dislodged by the blood pressure, which has returned to normal.

SECONDARY HAEMORRHAGE
Haemorrhage after seven to ten days. Bacterial infection can produce toxins, which may dissolve the clot.

THROMBOSIS
Thrombosis is the clotting of the blood in the blood vessels.

Aetiology
1. It occurs where the endothelium of the vessel has been damaged.
2. In many conditions the blood clots more readily, e.g. after trauma (including surgery).

Pathology
The damaged endothelium attracts platelets, which become attached to the damaged area. These then release enzymes causing the clot (thrombus) to form.

ARTERIAL THROMBOSIS
At the site of an injury or disease, such as an atheromatous plaque in aorta, femoral artery or coronary arteries.

Results
The distal blood supply to the limb or organ is severely diminished or cut off. If severe enough, this leads to its death (gangrene).

Treatment
1. Try to dissolve the clot with fibrin-dissolving enzymes—streptokinase (Kabinase, 100 000 i.u. hourly).
2. *Operation.* The artery is opened and the thrombus removed. If necessary, the damaged inner layer of the artery is also removed by endarterectomy (end = endothelium).
3. If it is long-standing, the blockage may be by-passed with a graft (p. 39).

VENOUS THROMBOSIS
It is most often seen in the leg veins.

Superficial venous thrombosis
Confined to the superficial veins of the leg and is often a complication of varicose veins (p. 42). The stasis leads to thrombus formation in the damaged veins.

Clinical features
The veins are very tender and feel like thin cord, and walking is painful.

Treatment
If very severe the patient should be rested until the inflammation subsides.
  Less severe cases can continue to be ambulant with firm bandaging to the leg.

Thrombo-phlebitis
Virtually the same as superficial thrombosis, but with very marked inflammation associated with the thrombosis.

Deep venous thrombosis
Thrombosis of the deep leg veins (p. 42) or pelvic veins. This is much more dangerous.

Clinical features
The blood has difficulty leaving the lower limb and oedema develops.
  Pain is felt in the calves and dorsiflexion of the foot and is painful.
  There may be *no* symptoms if the veins are only partially blocked.

Treatment
1. Anticoagulants to stop further thrombosis.
2. Complete bed rest for ten days is essential.
3. Supporting bandaging helps the oedema.

Complication
The thrombus may break free and form a thromboembolus (see below).

Embolus

An embolus is a foreign body in the blood stream.

Causes
1. Air (i.v. drip; cut throat) which may lead to an air lock in the heart and death (probably requires at least 25 ml in an adult).
2. Fat (from marrow after fractures) may block the pulmonary capillaries in the lungs and so cause anoxia.
3. Bacterial (from abscess) causes distant abscesses (p. 10).
4. Thromboembolus.

THROMBOEMBOLUS
The most important and most common. Starts as a thrombus which becomes detached from the wall.

ARTERIAL THROMBOEMBOLUS
Arterial thromboemboli travel distally until they try to enter too small an artery and so block it.

Result
Lack of blood (ischaemia) to the limb or organ which may die, causing for example gangrene of a limb or gangrene of the bowel.

Treatment
Embolectomy (removal of clot at operation) may be possible.

VENOUS THROMBOEMBOLUS
Venous thromboemboli arise mainly in pelvic or deep leg veins (p.42). The thrombus travels via the inferior vena cava and right side of the heart to the lung, where it blocks a pulmonary vessel too small for it to enter. It may be a massive embolus or a small one and in the lung is called a *pulmonary embolus*. A portion of lung may die as a result of the blocked artery (pulmonary infarct).

Symptoms
Depend on the size of the embolus.
1. If the embolus is large and blocks all blood to the lungs, the patient becomes cyanosed, gasping for breath and rapidly unconscious. Death quickly follows.
2. In less severe cases, there is sudden chest pain, especially with respiration.
3. The patient may be shocked, and even cyanosed.
4. Next day the sputum is blood flecked as a result of the pulmonary damage.

Treatment
1. Oxygen.
2. Try to dissolve the embolus with the enzyme streptokinase (p. 35).
3. Operation—try to remove clot—reserved for the most serious.

Methods of prevention
1. Early mobilisation after operation.
2. The calves of patients should be prevented from resting on the operating table, by using a heel rest.
Or
3. Use plastic bags which periodically inflate and deflate, massaging the legs during operation and so stopping venous stasis.
4. A low dose of heparin at the time of operation and afterwards markedly reduces the risk.

Atheroma

The fat, *cholesterol*, is deposited in the walls of arteries causing ulceration of the endothelium and narrowing of the lumen. Both animal fats, which are high in cholesterol, and smoking are thought to be part of the cause.

Result
1. A *thrombus* may form on the ulcers of the endothelium (p. 34).
2. An *aneurysm* may result from the weakening of the vessel allowing it to dilate.
3. *Vascular insufficiency* can develop as the build up of deposits gradually narrows the lumen and reduces the blood flow. In arteries to organs or limbs, if severe enough, it can lead to their death (arteriosclerotic gangrene).

ANEURYSM
An aneurysm is a sac connected to or part of an artery. It may be *congenital*, as in the case of the cerebral vessels (p. 147) or *acquired* from atherosclerosis, infection or trauma. Aneurysms of the thoracic and abdominal aorta are largely due to atheroma.

Pathology
The wall of the artery becomes weakened and the blood pressure pushes out the weakness. The aneurysm may be fusiform, saccular or dissecting.

A dissecting aneurysm of the aorta is the result of the blood rupturing through between the arterial coats at an atheromatous ulcer and dissecting them. They often end in complete rupture (see below).

ABDOMINAL AORTIC ANEURYSM
Clinical features
1. A pulsatile swelling in the midline which may by symptomless.
2. It may cause symptoms by pressing on organs or nerves.
3. The diagnosis is confirmed by aortogram (X-rays following the injection into the aorta of a radio opaque dye).

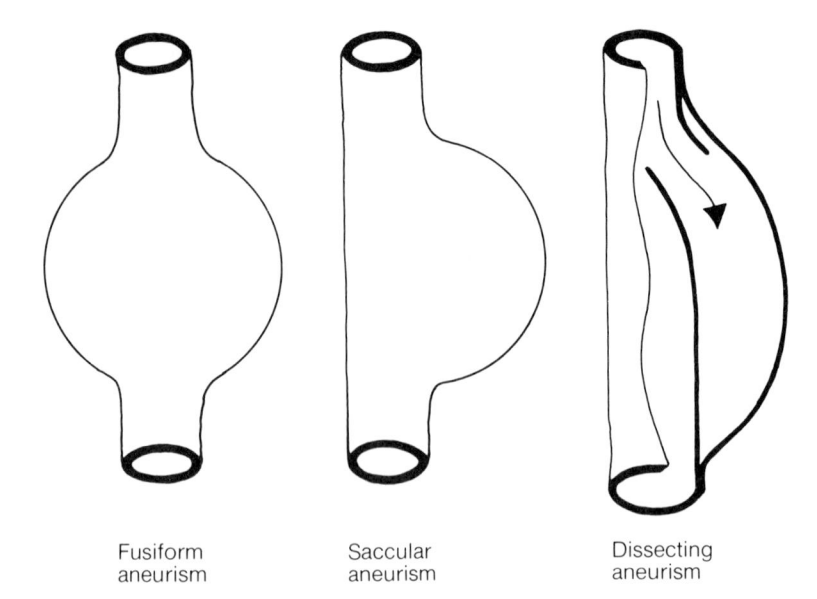

Figure 11.1
Blood and vascular disorders –
aneurism

Fusiform aneurism

Saccular aneurism

Dissecting aneurism

Treatment
Most are amenable to surgery. The aneurysm is replaced by a woven, artificial fibre graft, which is carefully stitched in place (p. 39).

RUPTURED AORTIC ANEURYSM
This is the usual fate of an untreated aneurysm. The rupture varies from a slow leak to a sudden massive haemorrhage.

Clinical features
They vary with the severity of the leak.
1. Abdominal pain which gradually gets worse.
2. Abdominal distension from the blood leak is associated with severe gastro-intestinal upsets.
3. Shock develops leading to death.
4. If a massive rupture, then these symptoms will lead to death in a few minutes.

Treatment
An attempt is made if possible to replace the ruptured aorta with a woven graft (p. 39). But the mortality is much higher than replacing an unruptured aneurysm.

VASCULAR INSUFFICIENCY
Vascular insufficiency, caused by progressive narrowing of the arterial lumen, leads to *anoxia* and *nutritional* changes in the organ supplied. Each part, however, will present with individual clinical features, e.g. angina pectoris from the cardiac anoxia, personality changes from cerebral anoxia.

The *lower limb* is commonly affected.

Clinical features
1. Loss of peripheral pulses and cold extremity.
2. Shiny, paper-thin skin and hyperkeratotic nails from lack of nutrition and anoxia.
3. Intermittent claudication—pain in the calves with exercise which causes an increased oxygen need that cannot be met (similar to cardiac angina).
4. In slowly progressive cases an alternative blood supply develops—collateral circulation which may protect the limb.
5. If the collateral circulation is insufficient then the part dies (gangrene).

Treatment
1. Stop smoking as it causes severe peripheral vasoconstriction making the situation worse.
2. Very great care must be taken of the limb to avoid injury or infection.
3. Exercise within the limit of the pain should be encouraged.
4. Arterial grafts may be possible to improve the blood supply.

Aortic and arterial grafts
These consist of:
1. Woven artificial fibre (Dacron, Terylene) grafts. These are obtained in two shapes, but many sizes.
   a. The long tube for arterial bypass or replacement, e.g. femoral artery.
   b. The inverted Y for aortic and common iliac artery replacement.

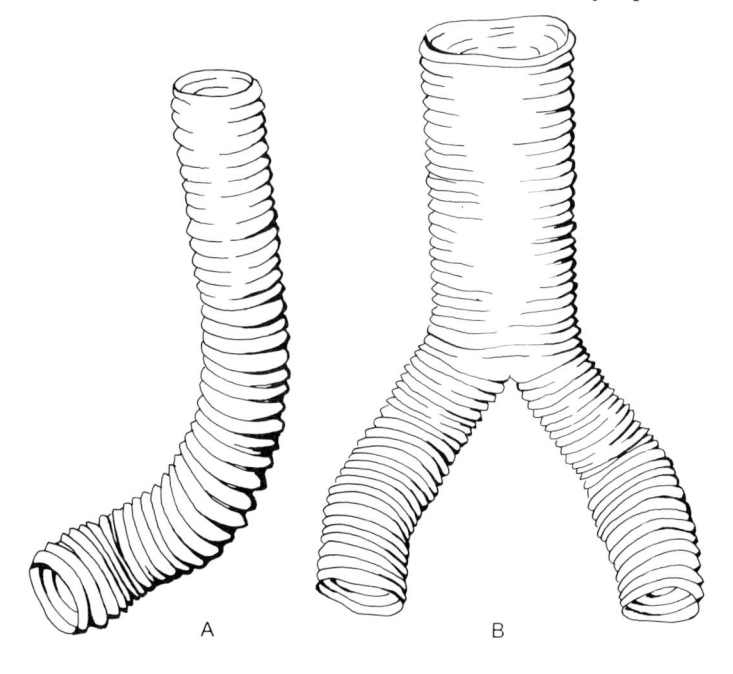

Figure 11.2
Terylene woven arterial grafts

A — Arterial by-pass

B — Inverted Y for aortic graft

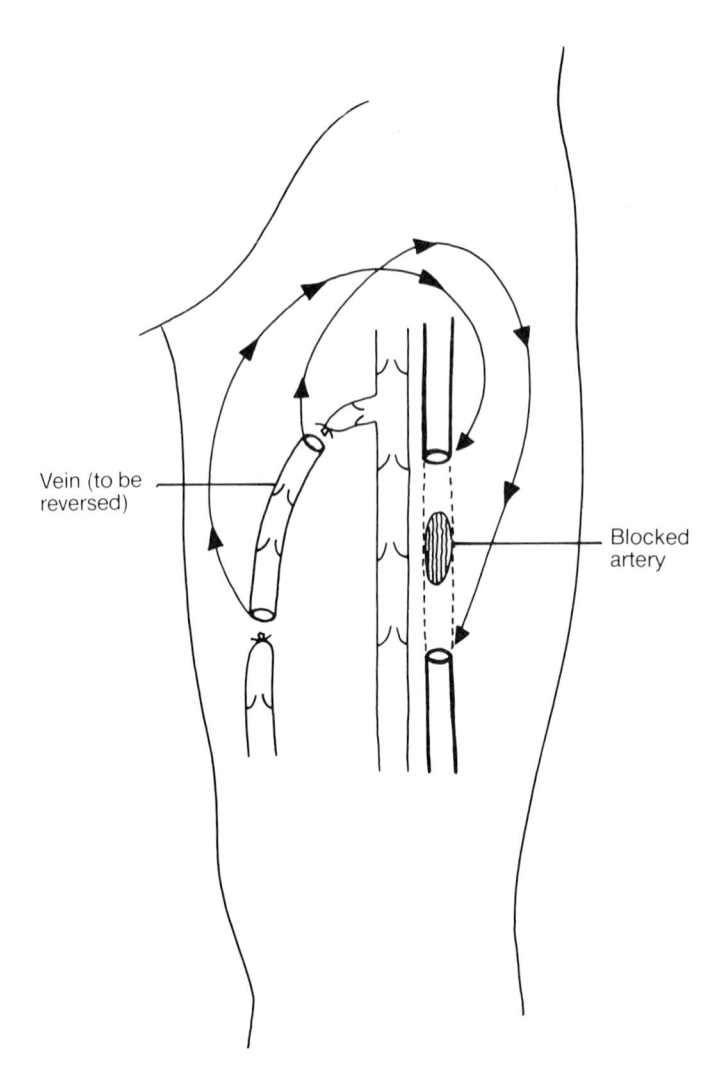

Figure 11.3
Superficial vein graft

2. Vein grafts are much less popular now the woven grafts are so good. A superficial leg vein is excised and used to by-pass the blocked limb artery. It has to be reversed because of the valves, i.e. distal end to proximal end of artery.

Gangrene

Death of a limb or organ of the body.

AETIOLOGY
1. *Injury*. Trauma damages the blood vessels, and the tissues which they supply die.
2. *Infective*. Boils, carbuncles show local gangrene (see also gas gangrene p. 13).
3. *Vascular*. The commonest causes of gangrene of the lower limbs are arteriosclerosis, thrombosis and embolism. But prolonged vessel

BLOOD AND VASCULAR DISORDERS

spasm seen in Ergot poisoning or Raynauds disease may lead to gangrene of the feet or hands.

CLINICAL FEATURES
1. There is no blood supply to the part (e.g. leg).
2. The skin changes colour becoming dark and even black.
3. If sudden, the tissues are normal and well hydrated, thus when dead they are easily infected and blisters form (wet gangrene).
4. If slow, the tissues gradually become dehydrated and wizened, and bacteria cannot invade them (dry gangrene).

TREATMENT
1. The limb is exposed to keep it cool and dry to encourage *dry* not *wet* gangrene, thus inhibiting infection.
2. Granulation tissue will form between the living and dead tissues, gradually separating them—the line of demarcation. When this is obvious then amputation is carried out.
3. Gangrene of the bowel (p. 118) is always *wet* gangrene and always requires *immediate surgery*.

Amputations

Amputations are carried out for:
1. Gangrene.
2. Malignant growths.
3. Injury.
4. Congenital deformity.

1. *Vascular gangrene* is often associated with poor blood supply so that a high amputation, well beyond the line of demarcation, is necessary. It invariably involves the lower limb, not the upper.

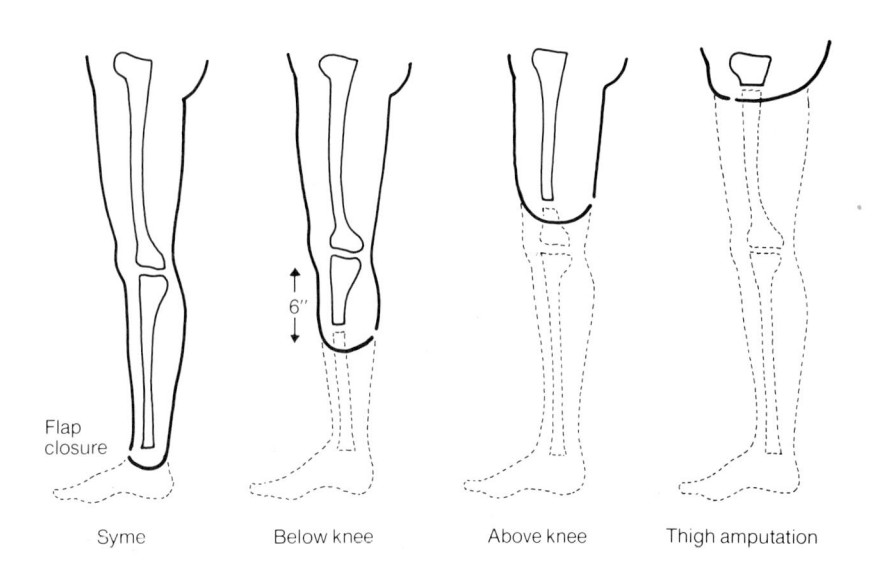

Figure 11.4 Amputation

Syme — Below knee — Above knee — Thigh amputation

2. *Malignant disease* may require a very radical amputation to remove the disease.
3. In *injury* as much of the limb is preserved as possible.
4. *Congenital deformity* is amputated only where it constitutes a nuisance to the patient.

EARLY POSTOPERATIVE TREATMENT
1. The stump is watched for infection and secondary haemorrhage.
2. Careful bandaging is essential to 'mould' the stump to a conical shape for easy fitting of an artificial limb.
3. Active exercises of the stump must be commenced early to maintain and strengthen the remaining muscles and to stop contractures forming at the joints.
4. Early ambulation and when the stump has healed the artificial limb is fitted.

VARICOSE VEINS

The veins in the legs are in two groups, *superficial veins* which lie immediately under the skin and *deep veins* which lie beside the arteries. Valves are present in the veins which ensure the blood flow is in one direction only, i.e. from the superficial vein through a *communicator* vein to a deep vein and to the inferior vena cava. If the valves are damaged, blood can flow back causing an increased pressure in the superficial veins and so dilating them, giving *varicose veins*.

Clinical features
1. The veins become dilated and tortuous, especially on standing.
2. There is often an aching tiredness in the legs, especially at night.

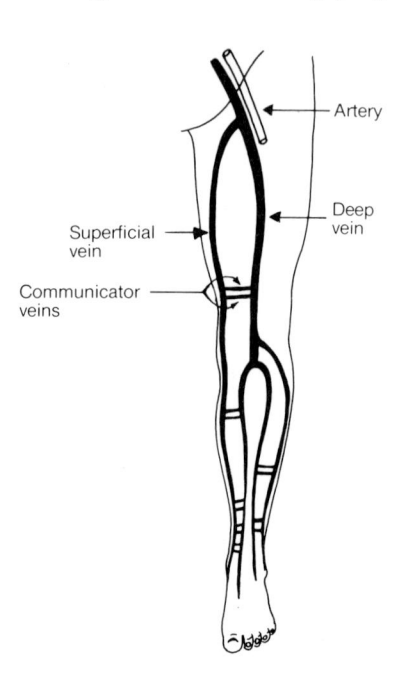

Figure 11.5
Varicose veins

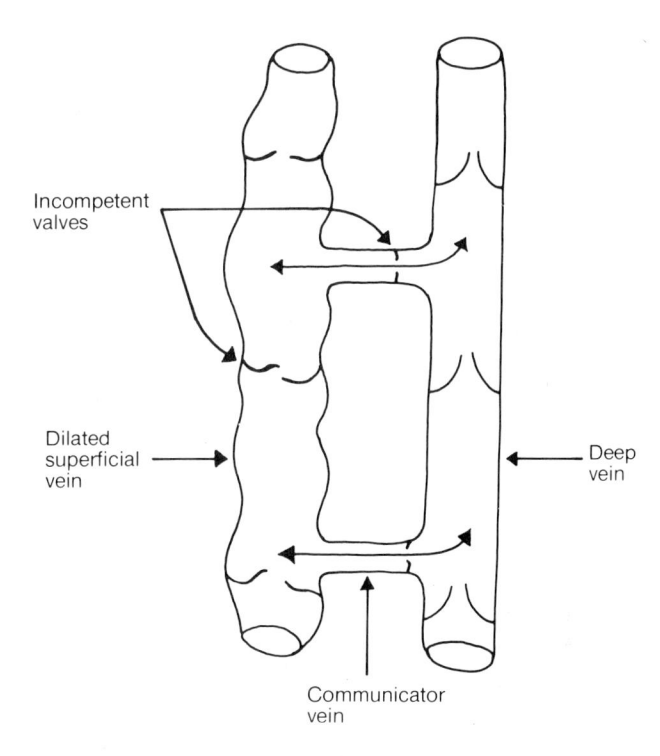

Figure 11.6
Varicose veins

Treatment
1. *Elastic stockings* gives support and stop the veins dilating, so forcing the blood into the deep veins.
2. *Injection.* Small varicose veins can be destroyed by injection of an irritant into the lumen. This causes a local inflammation that sticks the sides of the vein wall together—ethanolamine 2 ml.
3. *Ligation.* The veins are exposed at the damaged valves and ligated, thus stopping the back flow.
4. *Stripping.* Where the vein has many damaged valves and is grossly dilated it is totally removed or stripped.

Note: After the above procedures, the blood returns to the heart by the many other non-varicose veins.

VARICOSE ULCER
At the ankle the effect of the back pressure is most severe and it causes stasis in the venous drainage, and over the course of time venules may rupture leading to skin pigmentation. The tissues are chronically ill-nourished and anoxic. Their healing capacity is impaired and any slight injury may become an ulcer, which gradually enlarges.

Treatment
1. Remove the cause, i.e. the back pressure by counteracting it with elastic bandaging, or if necessary complete bed rest. (Elastic stockings and crepe bandaging do not have sufficient 'squeeze' in the treatment of an ulcer.

2. Once the above is achieved the ulcer heals quickly with simple dressings under the elastic bandage (Melonex).
3. When the ulcer is healed, the varicose veins are dealt with by operation.

VARICOSE ECZEMA
Before the ulcer actually forms the tissues may become infected and this causes a dermatitis.

Clinical features
1. The skin is reddened and oedematous.
2. There is severe itching.

Treatment
Treatment is the same as for ulcers using an anti-inflammatory dressing.

12 Skin

Infections

These are commoner where ill health is weakening the general resistance. Diabetics are especially at risk. All patients must therefore have their urine tested to exclude diabetes.

FURUNCLE (boil)
A staphylococcal infection of a hair follicle, which becomes a superficial abscess.

Treatment
1. Surgical incision relieves the pain, and a specimen of pus is taken for bacterial culture.
2. Antibiotics may be used to prevent spread. The choice of antibiotic depends on the culture.

CARBUNCLE
A staphylococcal infection involving a group of hair follicles, leading to abscess formation and necrosis of the skin.

Treatment
1. Antibiotics are used early to limit spread.
2. Incision and drainage of abscesses.

CYSTS

Sebaceous cyst
A cyst filled with sebum and epithelial developed from a sebaceous gland whose duct had become blocked. Present as a swelling usually on the scalp or face.

Treatment is surgical excision. They may become infected and require incision first and removal at a later date.

Inclusion dermoids

Epithelial or dermal cells may become buried (included) deep to the skin. Instead of dying, they multiply to form and eventually to line the wall of the cyst. The fluid content of the cyst is the result of the breakdown of desquamated cells. There are two types: implantation and congenital.

IMPLANTATION DERMOID
Commonly found in the hands where a piercing injury (e.g. from a needle) has driven epithelial cells into the subcutaneous tissues. They form a cyst which presents as a small, discrete swelling.

CONGENITAL DERMOID
In the embryo there are many places where skin tissues meet and fuse. Epithelial cells may become buried and survive to form a cyst in later life at these junction points, e.g. midline of back, from the spinal cord development (p. 151), in the neck and face from facial and maxillary fusion (p. 51).

Malignant tumours

SQUAMOUS CELL CARCINOMA (Epithelioma)
A malignant tumour of the skin that can be caused by prolonged exposure to sunlight and some chemicals, e.g. tar. It metastasises to the regional lymph glands.

Clinical features
1. Presents initially as a painless nodule which eventually becomes a typical malignant ulcer.
2. Enlarged lymph glands may be present. This is exemplified especially in carcinoma of the lip.

Treatment
1. Surgical excision or radiotherapy.
2. This is followed by radiotherapy to the draining lymph glands.

BASAL CELL CARCINOMA (rodent ulcer)
Arises from the basal cells of the skin, and is usually on the face. Common in countries where there is very strong sunlight. They do *not* metastasis, but present as a nodule which becomes an ulcer.

Treatment
Treatment is surgical excision or radiotherapy.

MALIGNANT MELANOMA
A very malignant tumour of the pigment cells of the skin. They spread early to the regional lymph glands.

Clinical features
1. A pigmented spot, which is growing, changing colour or bleeding.
2. There may be enlarged lymph nodes.

Treatment
1. Wide excision of the lesion.

2. Excision of the regional lymph glands (the tumour is resistant to radiotherapy).
3. Cytotoxics may be given for metastatic disease, but the the results are disappointing.

13 Plastic surgery

Plastic surgery repairs defects and injuries to the tissues of the body. Skin is the main tissue involved, with cartilage, blood vessels, and bone next in descending order of frequency.

Replacement of skin defects

The replacement of skin defects is carried out by two main methods, free skin grafts and skin flaps.

1. Free skin grafts. The skin is *completely detached* from the donor site and from its blood supply. Its survival depends on receiving enough nourishment and oxygen from the slight exudate at the grafted (recipient) site until capillaries grow into it. These grafts may be split skin (partial thickness) or full thickness grafts.

2. Skin flaps. The skin always remains *partially attached* and always has a blood supply. A flap of skin is raised (with the underlying tissue, if required) but left partially attached by a base or pedicle. The blood supply is thus maintained through the base until a new blood supply grows from the receiving area. This type of graft varies from the simple skin flap to the complex tubed pedicle graft.

Free skin grafts

SPLIT SKIN
This is the most common graft and can be used to cover large areas (e.g. after burns). It is taken from the healthy area (donor site) with a special knife. The thin sheet of skin is laid on the receiving area (recipient site)

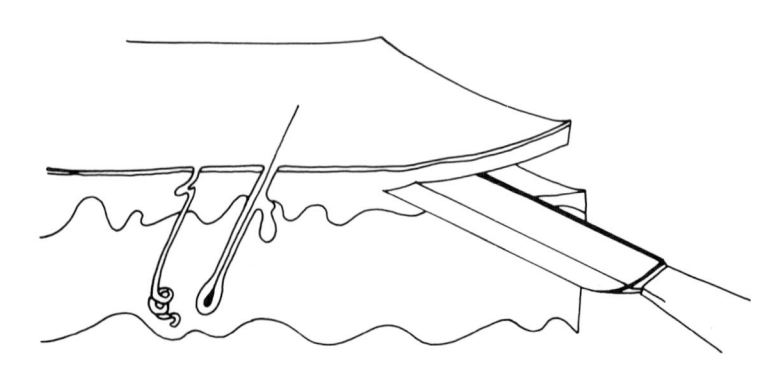

Figure 13.1
Split skin graft

and held there with dressings and stitches until capillaries and fibroblasts have grown in from below and secured it (ten days). The donor site heals by regenerating the remaining cells (as with superficial burns) and can even be used again for further grafts.

FULL THICKNESS GRAFT (Wolfe graft)

The full dermis with the basal layer is taken by excising with a knife. The graft is therefore of necessity small. The thickness of skin gives a much better texture and colour and is used on faces and hands. The donor area (any area where skin is loose, e.g. abdomen, forearm) is closed with stitches.

Skin flaps

Local flaps

These are flaps used to close defects locally. They depend partly on the stretching of the skin. The simplest is undercutting the edges of the wound to allow them to be drawn together with sutures. A defect can be closed by the advancement of a simple flap, or by the use of a V–Y flap.

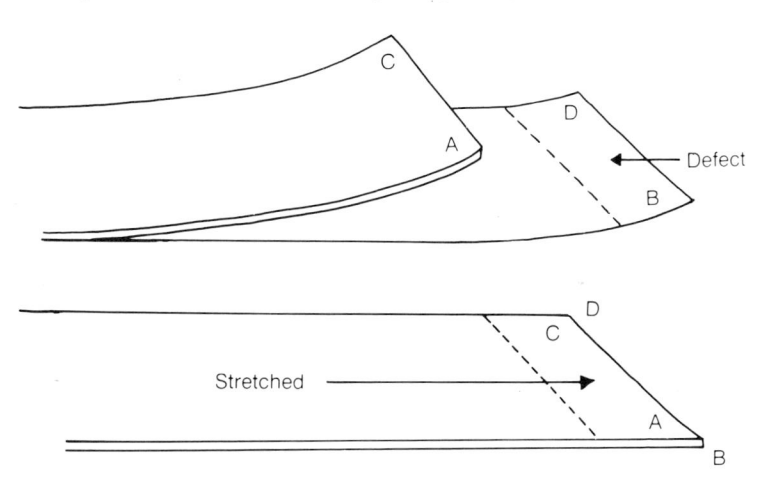

Figure 13.2
Full thickness local flap advancement

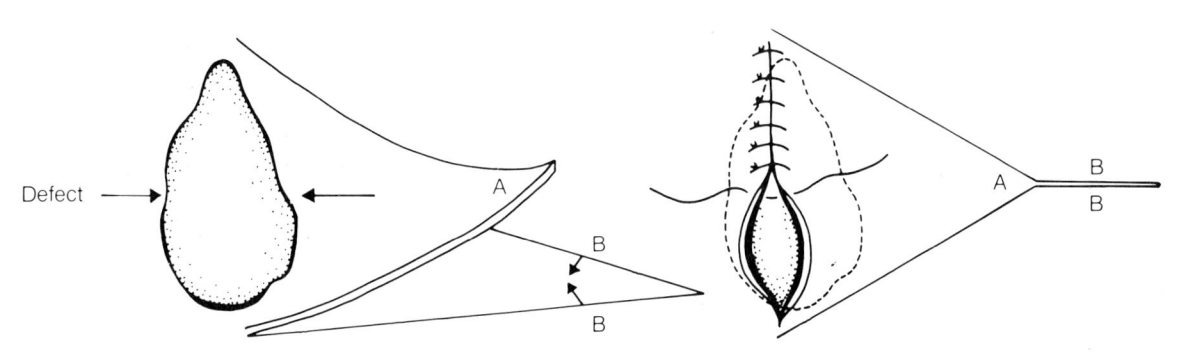

Figure 13.3
Full thickness local V–Y flap

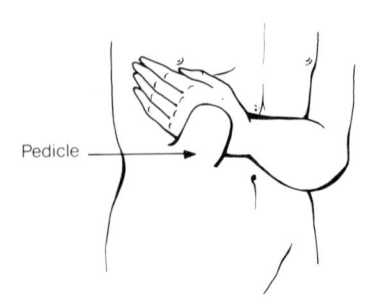

Figure 13.4
Direct pedicle graft

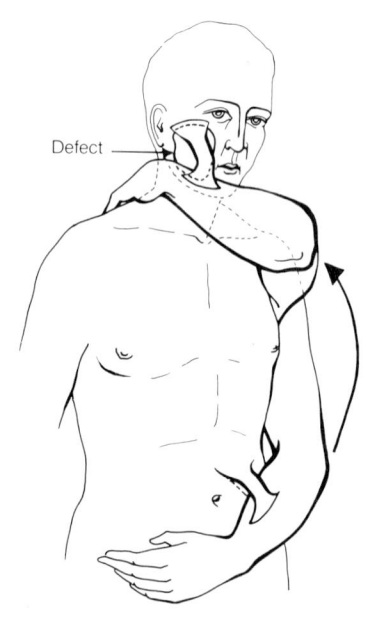

Figure 13.5
Tubed pedicle graft

PEDICLE GRAFTS

Direct pedicle graft

This skin flap can supply *directly* a full thickness graft to a limb by bringing the limb to the donor site, e.g. abdomen. The flap is raised and is attached to the edge of the receiving (recipient) area. Once new blood vessels grow in and supply it, the base can be detached from the donor site. The donor site is closed by sutures, or even a further split skin graft.

Tubed pedicle grafts

The aim is to move a pedicle graft to a distant part. A flap is raised, but turned into a tube and its free edge is then attached to an intermediate site, e.g. a limb, forearm. When a new blood supply from the limb is established it is *detached* from the original site. The limb is moved to the receiving area for the graft. The tube is opened and attached to the receiving area. After a new blood supply is established the graft is *detached from the limb*.

Cartilage and bone

Both of these are transplanted, e.g. a rib can be used to refashion a jaw bone and cavities in bone caused by disease can be filled with bone chips removed from the ileum. Costal cartilage can be used to model the cartilage of the nose where this has been destroyed (for blood vessels see p. 39).

Blood Vessels See p. 39

Different types of grafts

AUTOGRAFTS

All those described above are autografts. The tissues used are taken from the patient.

HOMOGRAFT

These tissues used are from another human being and they will be reject them as suppressed by drugs e.g. steroids and azathioprine (Imuran). Corneal grafting of the eye is another example, but it is not rejected, as the immunity response in the cornea, which has no blood supply, is so weak.

Kidney transplants are homografts and the immunity which would reject them is suppressed by drugs. Steroids and azathioprine (Imuran). Corneal grafting of the eye is another example, but it is not rejected, as the immunity response in the cornea, which has no blood supply, is so weak.

HETEROGRAFTS (Zenografts)

These are materials unrelated to humans. Terylene grafts are used for aortas. Animal tissues such as bone or pig skin (p. 24) are also used.

14 Head and neck

Embryology

The primary oral orifice is modified into the mouth and nose by lateral maxillary processes which form and then grow medially. The palate and upper lip are formed by the maxillary processes meeting a nasal process, which grows down. Failure of the growing maxillary and nasal bones to grow together and fuse causes gaps or 'clefts' to remain.

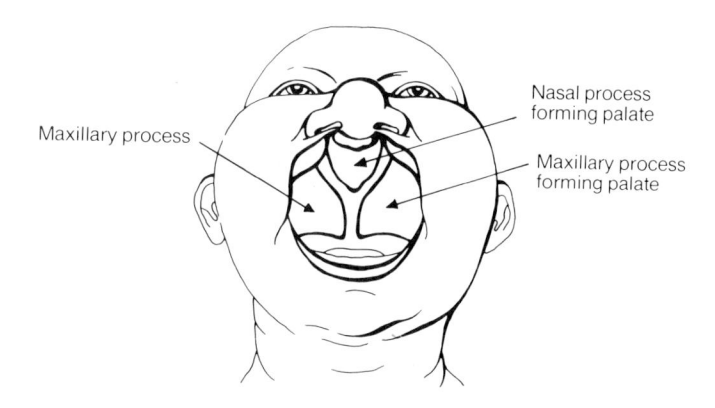

Figure 14.1
Type of cleft palate (tripartite) with double cleft lip

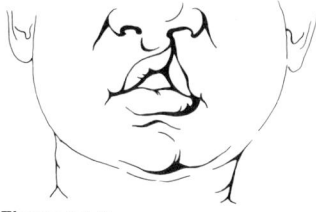

Figure 14.2
Cleft lip

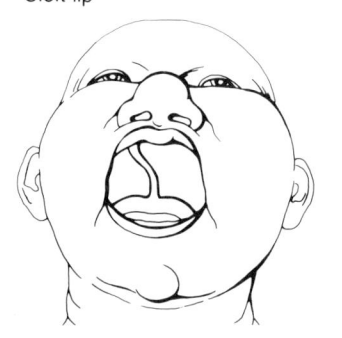

Figure 14.3
Type of cleft palate (bipartite)

CLEFT (HARE) LIP
A split which may stretch from the upper lip to the nostril. Occasionally it is bilateral.

Treatment
A very careful plastic repair is carried out at age three to six months.

CLEFT PALATE
The lateral parts of the palate fail to meet either with the nasal process or with each other and fuse in the midline (giving a tripartite or bipartite cleft). The mouth thus communicates with the nasal cavity. A minor degree involves the soft palate only.

Clinical features
1. The child has difficulty sucking and swallowing.
2. Food enters the nose.
3. If the deformity is not corrected, the speech is badly affected and there is a marked dental deformity.

Treatment
Very careful closure is carried out in the first year of life.
The majority of patients have a combined cleft lip and cleft palate.

MOUTH

STOMATITIS
Inflammation of the mouth, with red, painful mucous membrane, which may become ulcerated.

Causes
Bacterial, fungal or viral infection.

Bacterial
Certain bacteria cause an acute inflammation often with bleeding gum (Vincents Angina). It is very contagious.

Treatment. Penicillin orally.

Fungal (Candida albicans).
An infection seen as white patches on the mucous membrane (thrush). Common in young children or in adults after prolonged antibiotic therapy.

Treatment. Nystatin mouth washes quickly clear it.

Viral
Seen in measles (Koplik's spots). It is very transient.

Other causes of stomatitis
Other causes of stomatitis include trauma, burns, chemicals, drugs and vitamin deficiencies.

APHTHOUS ULCER
An acute very painful ulcer of the mucous membrane. The aetiology is unknown. It heals spontaneously after several days, with no scarring. But a few patients develop recurrent ulceration, which eventually causes scarring and contraction of the mucous membrane. There is no real treatment of benefit. Mouth washes may soothe the ulcers.

MALIGNANT ULCERS
Most common on the lip and tongue (see below), but may develop elsewhere, such as on the cheek or below the tongue. Presents as a painless ulcer with a thickened edge.
   Treatment is surgical excision of the ulcer with radiotherapy to the related lymph glands.

Tongue

GLOSSITIS
Inflammation of the tongue. The aetiology is the same as for stomatitis.

TONGUE TIE
A congenital short fraenum or frenulum anchors the tongue to the floor of the mouth.

Clinical features
1. Baby may have difficulty in sucking.
2. Speech is affected later.

Treatment
Simple division frees the tongue.

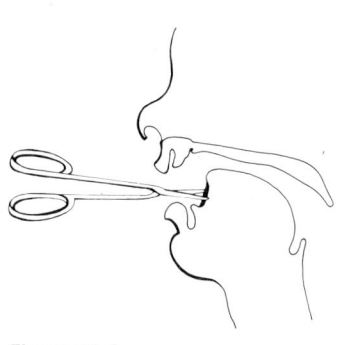

Figure 14.4 Division of frenulum in tongue tie

ULCERS OF THE TONGUE

Simple ulcers
Usually caused by trauma from a carious tooth or badly fitting denture.

MALIGNANT ULCER (Squamous cell carcinoma)
Found mostly at the side of the tongue in elderly men. Chronic irritation (e.g. pipe smoking) predisposes to it.

Clinical features
1. A raised *ulcer* with a thickened edge.
2. It is *painless*.
3. The ulceration causes *bad breath* (halitosis).
4. Eventually there is difficulty in eating and swallowing.

Treatment
1. If possible, *surgical excision* of the primary tumour with radiotherapy to the draining cervical lymph glands.
2. If inaccessible (back of tongue) or too large, then *radiotherapy* alone is used.

The lip

HERPES SIMPLEX (Cold sore)
A recurrent acute blistering of the lip, caused by a virus of the same name, which becomes crusted after a few days and heals with no scarring.

Treatment
Dry it with surgical spirit. 'Herpid' an antiviral drug applied locally may clear it quickly.

CHANCRE OF LIP
Primary syphilitic lesion. A small painless ulcer. Heals after two to three weeks with little scarring.

Treatment
As for syphilis.

CARCINOMA OF LIP (SQUAMOUS CELL)
Usually seen in men over sixty years. Chronic irritation (e.g. clay pipe smoking) can predispose to it.

Clinical features
An enlarging painless ulcer of the lip with hard thickened edge.

Treatment
1. *Surgical excision* through all the lip.
2. If thought necessary *radiotherapy* to the lymph glands of the neck.

LEUCOPLAKIA
A pre-malignant condition which presents on mucous membrane as white plaques. It is symptomless. It may take years to turn malignant. Found in the mouth and also in the oesophagus and vagina.

Treatment
Treatment is by *surgical excision*.

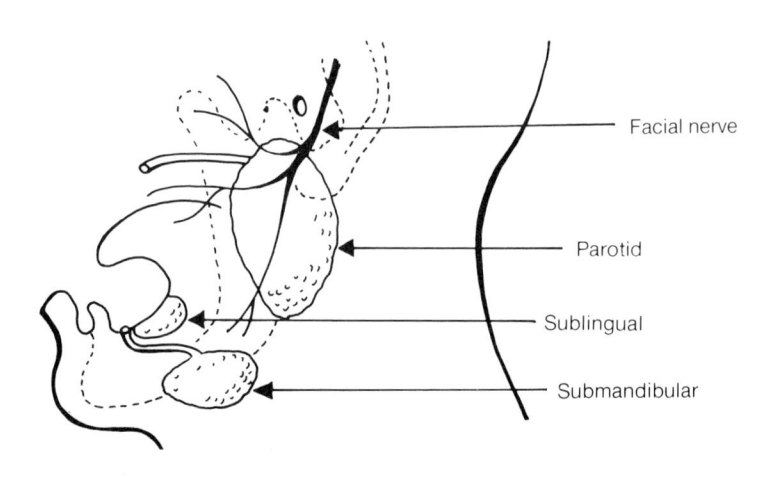

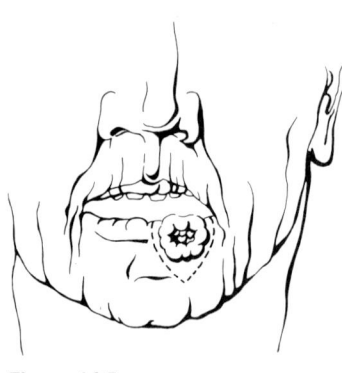

Figure 14.5 Carcinoma of the lip (malignant ulcer)

Salivary glands

There are three pairs of salivary glands:

1. *The parotid gland* is about two inches long and is situated behind the angle of the jaw below the ear. The parotid duct opens into the cheek opposite the second upper molar tooth. The facial nerve passes through the gland.

Figure 14.6 Salivary glands

2. *The submandibular gland* is tucked behind the jaw bone with the submandibular duct running across the floor of the mouth to open at the side of the frenulum.

3. *The sublingual gland* lies under the mucous membrane of the floor of the mouth lateral to the frenulum. It drains by many ducts to the floor of the mouth.

ACUTE PAROTITIS
Inflammation of the parotid gland.

Causes

Viral
Mumps, which in adults may very occasionally affect the pancreas and testes at the same time. It settles spontaneously.

Clinical features
Swelling and tenderness of one or both glands associated with a moderate general malaise.

Bacterial
Mainly in debilitated patients or post-operatively where there is dehydration coupled with poor oral hygiene. The staphylococcus is the usual bacteria.

Clinical features
1. Acutely tender and swollen parotid gland.
2. There is marked pyrexia.
3. The patient is markedly toxic.

Treatment
1. Antibiotics are given immediately.
2. If an abscess forms it is drained with care to avoid the facial nerve.

CHRONIC PAROTITIS
Presents as a tender, swollen gland. pressure on the gland produces pus from the duct.

Treatment
Treatment is a course of antibiotics and the routine emptying of the pus from the gland by gentle massage.
   Stimulating the gland to secrete and so wash itself clear is helpful and is achieved by regular sipping of unsweetened lemon juice.
   Inflammation of the other salivary glands is very rare.

SALIVARY CALCULUS
Collection of calcium and phosphates from tiny stones in gland or duct, usually in the submandibular, but occasionally in the parotid.

Clinical features
1. Calculi may block the duct and the gland, when stimulated by eating, becomes painful and swollen with secretion.
2. The swelling subsides after two to three hours.

Treatment
Surgical removal of the calculus.

Tumours of salivary glands

BENIGN
Mixed cell tumour—Arises as an adenoma with a mixture of cell types. Most commonly in the parotid.

Clinical features
A painless, very slow growing swelling of the salivary gland, which may become quite large.

Treatment
Surgical excision of the tumour is carried out taking a cuff of surrounding healthy tissue.

MALIGNANT
Carcinoma. Fairly rare.

Clinical features
A much quicker growing swelling, which is painless until it invades nerves.

Treatment
Total excision of the salivary gland. In the case of the parotid, this can lead to the excision of the facial nerve, which runs through the gland with resultant facial paralysis on that side.

Branchial cyst

A cyst arising from embrionic remnants in the side of the neck. It is often mistaken for enlarged lymph glands.

Clinical features
1. A discrete swelling below and behind the angle of the jaw appearing in early adult life.
2. It may become inflamed and painful.

Treatment
Surgical excision of the cyst.

Thyroglossal cyst

A cyst can develop from the remnants of embryonic tissue situated in the midline of the neck.

It presents as a discrete midline swelling usually close to the isthmus of the thyroid. Sometimes present at birth, but most appear in early adult life.

Treatment
Surgical excision of the cyst.

15 Thyroid gland

The thyroid gland consists of two lobes joined by an isthmus. They lie on the sides of the trachea just below the thyroid cartilage. The gland is formed by many follicles containing colloid. Surrounding the follicles are the parafollicular cells. It is controlled by the pituitary gland through its hormone TSH (thyroid stimulating hormone). It is an endocrine gland and secretes two hormones.

1. *Thyroxin* (contains iodine). Stimulates metabolism. It is made by the follicles.
2. *Calcitonin*. Regulates calcium metabolism and bone formation (partly in conjunction with parathormone p. 61). It is made by the parafollicular cells.

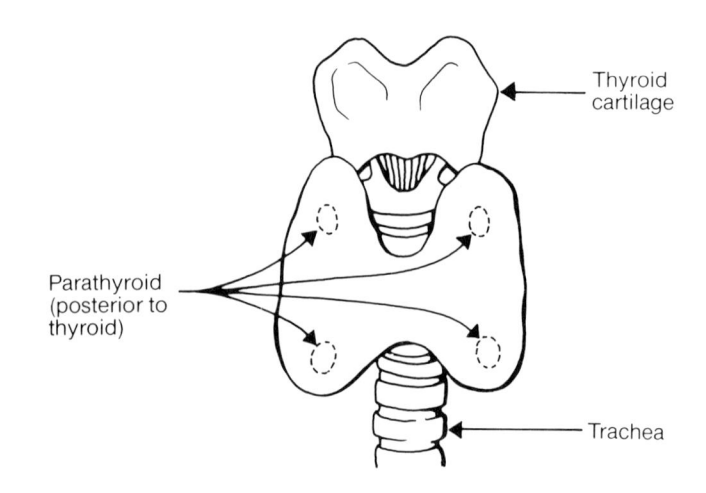

Figure 15.1
Thyroid gland

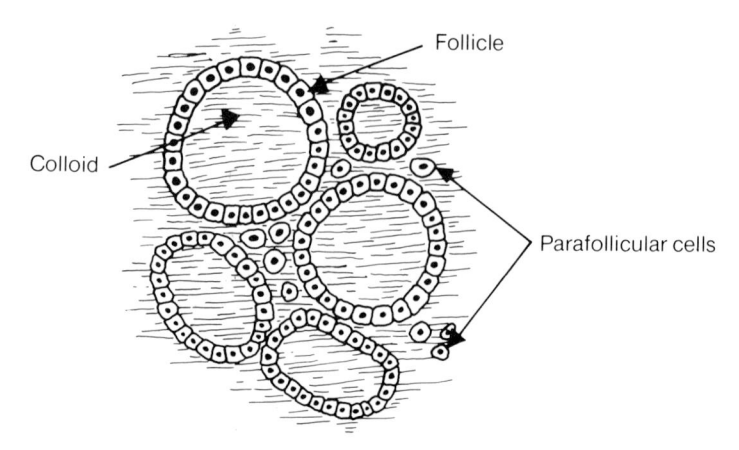

Figure 15.2
Colloid goitre

Goitre

Enlargement of the thyroid gland, due usually to the follicles over filling with colloid, and so it is often called *colloid goitre*. After years some of the follicles grow much larger forming cysts and the gland becomes nodular—*nodular goitre*. It is caused by a relative lack of iodine in the diet.

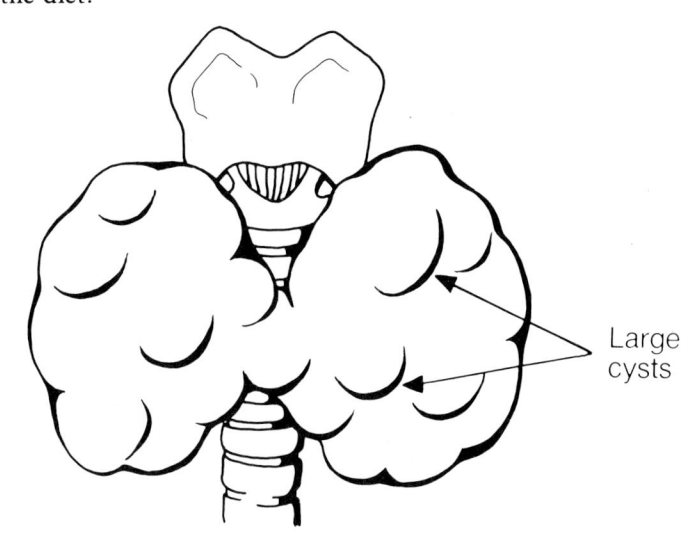

Figure 15.3
Nodular goitre

Clinical features
1. Thyroid gland is visibly and palpably enlarged.
2. There may be dysphagia and dyspnoea from pressure on oesophagus and trachea.

TREATMENT
Surgical excision (partial thyroidectomy).

Thyrotoxicosis

PRIMARY THYROTOXICOSIS
An overactive thyroid producing too much thyroxin.

SECONDARY THYROTOXICOSIS
A thyroid which is already a *goitre* and then becomes *thyrotoxic*.

CLINICAL FEATURES
1. Increased metabolism causes a hyperactive patient with an increased pulse rate, tolerance of cold.
2. There is loss of weight, but a good appetite.
3. The eyes become prominent—*exophthalmos*.
4. There is a fine tremor of the fingers and the palms are warm and moist.
5. The patients are often excitable and nervous and complain of sleeplessness.

Treatment

1. *Medical.* Antithyroid drugs, block the utilisation of iodine by the gland (Carbimazole 30 mg/day) and if they fail surgical treatment may be necessary.

2. *Surgery.* Partial thyroidectomy (removal of three quarters of the gland)

or

3. *Radioactive iodine.* It destroys the gland by local radiation when it is taken up by the gland and concentrated in the follicles. It is used only in older patients.

Tumours

BENIGN—ADENOMA
A solitary swelling in one lobe, with no other symptom.

Treatment
Treatment is surgical excision.

THYROID CYST
These are often adenomas which have degenerated and formed cysts. They may quickly enlarge as haemorrhage may occur into them. Presentation and treatment is the same as for adenoma.

CARCINOMA OF THYROID
It occurs more frequently in existing goitres.

Clinical features
1. *Hard swelling* in a thyroid lobe increasing in size.
2. It becomes *fixed* to the surrounding tissues.
3. It may cause *dysphagia* and *dyspnoea* by pressure.
4. There may be *hoarseness* if the vocal nerves are involved.

Treatment
1. Surgery. Total thyroidectomy, followed by radiotherapy.
2. Palliation, if very advanced, by radiotherapy alone.

HASHIMOTO'S DISEASE
The thyroid is gradually replaced by lymphocytes and fibrous tissue. The patient becomes hypothyroid. It is thought to be an auto-immune disease.

Treatment
Thyroxin 1 mg/day replacement.

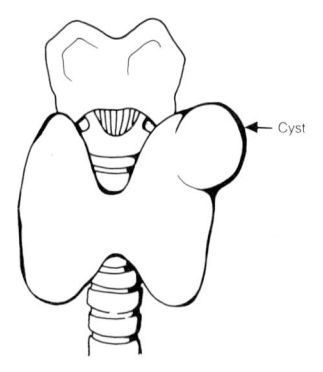

Figure 15.4 Thyroid cyst

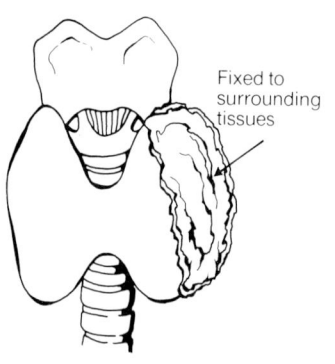

Figure 15.5 Carcinoma of thyroid

Parathyroid glands

Four tiny endocrine glands lying posterior to the lobes of the thyroid gland (p. 58). They produce *parathromone* which regulates the level of calcium and phosphorus in the blood.

HYPERPARATHYROIDISM
May be due to
1. Overactive glands (hyperplasia).
2. Benign tumour of one of the glands.

The increased hormone raises blood levels of calcium and phosphorus by taking it from the bones. It is then excreted in the urine.

Clinical features
1. There may be fractures due to weakening of the bones.
2. Renal calculi form due to increased excretion of calcium.

Treatment
Surgical excision of the tumour or in hyperplasia removal of three of the four glands.

HYPOPARATHYROIDSIM
The glands may be injured or accidentally removed at thyroidectomy. There is a fall in the calcium in the blood, which leads to muscle spasms (tetany). The fall is temporary with injury, but permanent with total removal (very rare).

Clinical features
1. SPASM of hands and feet (carpo-pedal).
2. Muscle cramps.
3. Feeling of suffocation.

Treatment
1. Intravenous calcium gluconate immediately (raises the serum calcium level).
2. Daily vitamin D and oral calcium keeps the blood level of calcium satisfactory in permanently injured cases or until the gland functions again.

16 Pharynx

The pharynx is a muscular tube, lined with squamous epithelium, connecting the *nose and mouth* to the *larynx and oesophagus*. The pharyngotympanic (Eustachian) tube from the middle ear enters the side wall above and behind the palate. Collections of lymphoid tissue are found in the pharyngeal wall; the *tonsil* lies in the side wall posterior to the tongue and the *adenoids* in the posterior wall, posterior to the

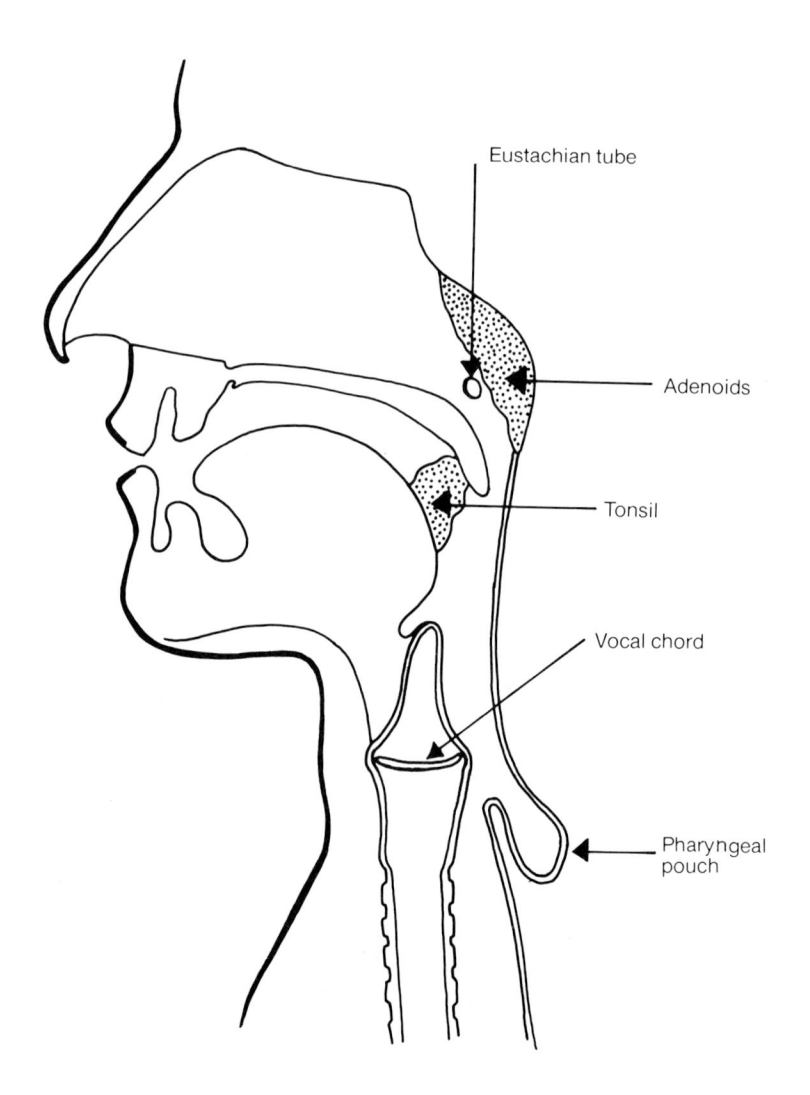

Figure 16.1
Pharynx

nose. It is described as being in three parts, nasopharynx, oropharynx and a laryngopharynx. A bolus of food or drink is swallowed by being pushed by the *tongue* against the *soft palate*. This stimulates the muscular contractions, which squeeze the bolus on to the oesophagus. Simultaneously to ensure nothing enters them, muscular contractions cause the palate to block the entrance to the nasopharynx and the epiglottis closes off the larynx.

Pharyngitis

Generalised inflammation most often caused by *viruses* (colds) or *bacteria* (Streptococcus).

Clinical features are a sore throat and general malaise. Most cases resolve without specific treatment.

Acute tonsillitis

The tonsils often become infected, especially in the child, either alone or with a pharyngitis. The commonest cause is a virus, but there may be a superimposed streptococcal infection.

CLINICAL FEATURES
1. The tonsils are inflamed, often with debris and pus on the surface.
2. Swallowing becomes painful.
3. There is often pyrexia.
4. Commonly the draining cervical glands are enlarged.

Most require no specific treatment, but if a streptococcal infection is present penicillin is given.

Chronic tonsillitis

The tonsil may become chronically infected.

CLINICAL FEATURES
1. Repeated exacerbations of acute tonsillitis (see above).
2. In the child the tonsils may become generally enlarged (hypertrophied).
3. The adult glands are often small and shrunken, but inflamed.

TREATMENT

Tonsillectomy
In the child this is usually a simple excision of the main hypertrophied portion (guillotine operation). In the adult the gland is totally removed by careful dissection.

Hypertrophy of tonsils and adenoids

TONSILS
Enlargement of the tonsils is common in children without infection being present. They usually cause no symptoms, but in very young children extreme enlargement may result in dysphagia and nasal obstruction. At puberty the glands shrink to the normal size.

ADENOIDS
These too may hypertrophy in the child, but they can cause symptoms by blockage of the nose and eustachian tubes.

Clinical features
1. Chronic nasal discharge causing snoring in the child.
2. Mouth breathing.
3. Recurrent otitis media (p. 69).

Treatment
Surgical removal by *adenoidectomy*.

Peritonsillar abscess (Quinsy)

An abscess which develops adjacent to the tonsil in the soft palate. The infection may have spread from the tonsil.

CLINICAL FEATURES
1. Severe pain in the throat especially on swallowing.
2. The mouth can only open a little and the patient is acutely ill.
3. The abscess bulges between the soft palate and tonsil displacing the uvula to the other side.

TREATMENT
1. Initially antibiotics may abort the infection.
2. Should an abscess form, it must be incised.

Pharyngeal pouch (see Fig. 16.1)

A diverticulum which develops in the laryngeal pharynx, probably as a result of disordered peristalsis. Food tends to enter it and it gradually enlarges. They may be symptomless, or there may be a gurgling in the neck on swallowing liquids. Large pouches on distension with food can cause severe dysphagia by pressing on the oesophagus.

Patients may learn to empty the pouch by pressing over it, but the treatment of choice is surgical excision.

Tumours

BENIGN
Pharyngeal tumours are rare.

CARCINOMA

The great majority (75 per cent) present with enlargement of the draining cervical glands due to metastases. Other symptoms, which are often late in appearing depend on the site.

NASOPHARYNGEAL

May cause nose bleeding (epistaxis) and nasal obstruction, with involvement of the eustachian tube, resulting in deafness.

OROPHARYNGEAL

May result in a persistently sore throat, blood stained sputum and halitosis (bad breath).

LARYNGOPHARYNGEAL

Often have minimal symptoms until quite advanced, when a persistently sore throat or dysphagia may develop.

Treatment

Depends on the site and the extent and consists of surgical excision or radiotherapy, or both.

Larynx

This is the 'voice box' and its lateral walls are formed mainly by the thyroid cartilages (Adams apple). It is continuous with the oropharynx above and the trachea below. The internal muscle (vocalis) covered by epithelium forms the vocal cords.

Laryngitis

There is a general inflammation from the same causes as pharyngitis. The voice may become hoarse or even lost from oedema of the vocal cords.

Tumours

BENIGN–PAPILLOMA

They develop usually on the vocal cords. Patient becomes hoarse. They are excised.

MALIGNANT—CARCINOMA: SQUAMOUS

Arise usually on the vocal cords. Patient becomes hoarse.

Treatment
1. Radiotherapy is the treatment of choice.
2. Surgical excision (laryngectomy) is reserved for recurrence. The distal trachea brought to the surface as a tracheostomy (tracheostome).

After laryngectomy the patient is unable to speak. Patients learn to speak by belching swallowed air from their stomachs as they mouth the words (oesophageal speech). Mechanical aids are also available.

LARYNGEAL PARALYSIS (Paralysis of the vocal cords)

Each cord is controlled by a recurrent laryngeal nerve, which runs upwards in the groove between trachea and oesophagus, on the left from the arch of the aorta in the thorax and on the right from the subclavian artery. One or both may be damaged by operation or invaded by tumour (p. 84).

Clinical features
1. The patient is hoarse and cannot cough properly (bovine cough).
2. Swallowing liquids may cause choking.
3. Unilateral paralysis is compensated by the other cord.
4. Bilateral paralysis is very serious and can cause dyspnoea and even death.

Treatment
If necessary, a tracheostomy and treatment of the cause.

Tracheostomy

An artificial opening in the trachea to help respiration.

REASONS FOR OPERATION

Emergency temporary
1. Because of an acute blockage of the upper airway, e.g. oedema, foreign body, laryngeal infection or bilateral laryngeal paralysis.
2. To allow positive pressure respiration.
   a. for chest injuries (p. 79)
   b. for diseases which cause paralysis (poliomyelitis) and others that require paralysis of the respiratory muscles (p. tetanus).
3. Occasionally persistent excessive bronchial secretions require a tracheostomy for their removal.

Permanent
After laryngectomy—*tracheostome* where the distal end is brought to the surface.

METHOD
The trachea is opened by cutting the cartilaginous rings and in emergency cases a soft plastic tube is inserted with an inflatable cuff, which makes a seal.

When the cuffed plastic tube is removed, the tracheostomy closes spontaneously.

In permanent cases, a silver tube is used.

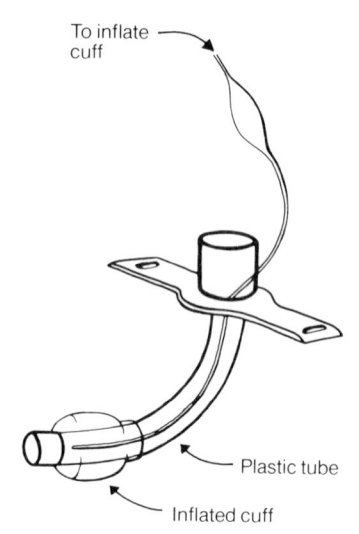

Figure 16.2
Tracheostomy cuff

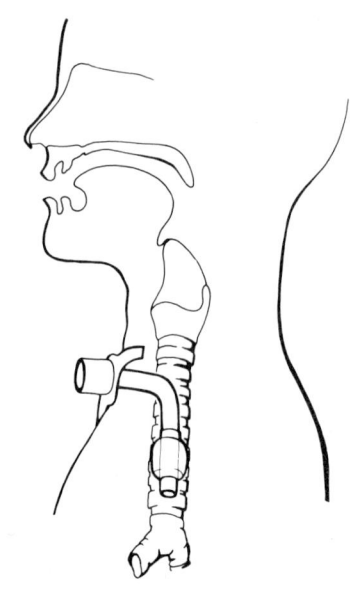

Figure 16.3
Tracheostomy

Ear

The ear consists of three parts.

The external ear consists of the pinna formed of cartilage which is closely attached to the skin. The pinna gathers the sound and funnels it into the external auditory canal. This canal lined by squamous epithelium is closed at the medial end by the tympanic membrane (ear drum) which is part of the middle ear.

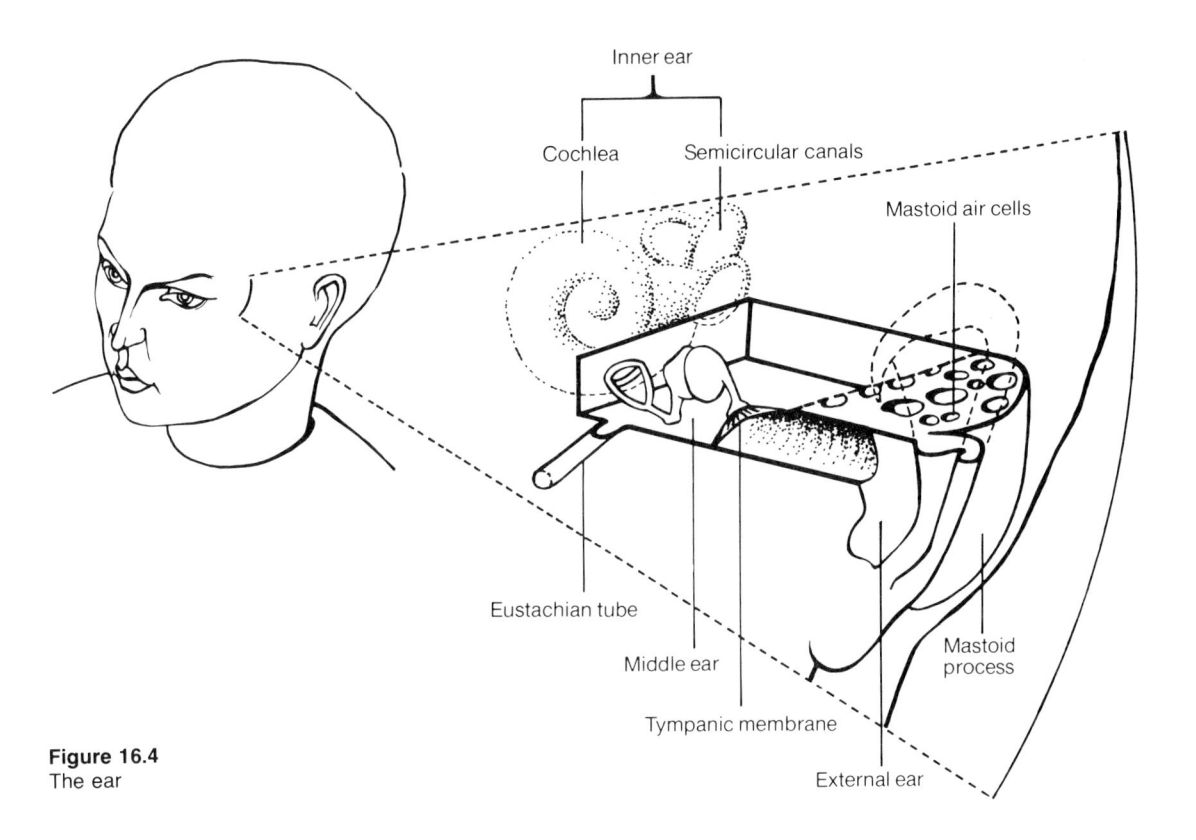

Figure 16.4
The ear

The middle ear accommodates the ossicles which transmit the vibration of the tympanic membrane to the inner ear. The middle ear is hollow, communicating with the pharynx by the pharyngotympanic tube and also with the air cells of the mastoid bone.

The inner ear is formed by the cochlea, which transmits the sounds to the auditory nerve and the semicircular canals, which in turn control balance.

BAT EARS
A congenital condition where the ears stick out. An operation which lessens their protrusion may be carried out for cosmetic purposes.

CARCINOMA OF THE PINNA (squamous cell carcinoma or rodent ulcer)
Presents as a malignant ulcer of the skin.

Treatment
Surgical excision through the full thickness of the pinna. After excision of a large malignancy, plastic surgical reconstruction of a new pinna may be necessary.

OTITIS EXTERNA
Inflammation of the external auditory meatus.

Aetiology
1. Due to infection causing an allergic inflammation.
2. The infection is secondary to the irritation produced by debris such as soap accumulations and dandruff.
3. Over-use of steroids, to treat the above may lead to a fungal infection.

Clinical features
1. There is a watery discharge associated with a severe irritation and itch.
2. The patient complains of deafness.

Treatment
1. Regular aural toilet.
2. Judicious use of ear drops containing a steroid plus an antibiotic.
3. A secondary fungal infection may require antifungal medication.

WAX
Some patients, due to a narrow opening, accumulate wax which forms a plug in the external auditory canal leading to deafness.

Treatment
Treatment consists of softening of the wax with oil, followed by its removal by gentle syringing.

SECRETORY OTITIS MEDIA
A condition usually limited to children.

The Eustachian tube becomes blocked, usually by adenoids (p. 64), so stopping the drainage of the middle ear.

An exudate builds up in the middle ear, at first it is watery, but it eventually becomes thick and glue-like (glue ear).

The exact cause of the exudate is often in doubt. It may be the end result of a bacterial otitis media treated by antibiotics, an allergic reaction, or a viral infection.

Clinical features
1. The child is deaf in that ear.

2. There is bulging of the drum, which has lost its glistening appearance and becomes lustreless.

Treatment
1. Incision of the drum (myringotomy) and drainage.
2. Adenoidectomy is also routinely carried out.

OTITIS MEDIA
Inflammation of the middle ear often secondary to an upper respiratory infection and enlarged adenoids. It is most common in children.

Clinical features
1. The child complains of severe pain in the ear.
2. There may be deafness.
3. It is often associated with pyrexia and in infants can cause convulsions.

Treatment
1. Early antibiotics usually cure it, plus nasal decongestants (ephedrine drops 0·5 per cent).
2. Adenoidectomy later if required.

Complications of otitis media

Acute mastoiditis
Spread of the infection in otitis media to the mastoid air cells, which become filled with pus.

Clinical features. (1) Symptoms of otitis media. (2) Pain and swelling over mastoid bone.

Treatment. (1) The vast majority respond to antibiotics. (2) If pus forms and it becomes chronic then part of the mastoid process is excised to allow drainage (Mastoidectomy).

Intracranial infections
Have become rare complications because of the benefit of antibiotics.

LABYRINTHITIS
Inflammation of the *inner ear*. It may be secondary to otitis media, but most are caused by viral infections and spontaneously resolve.

The patient complains of acute giddiness unless prone and also deafness, which can become permanent. Severe, prolonged vomiting may be a feature, and the patient has a 'flu' like illness. If secondary to otitis media, then antibiotics are required.

Menieres syndrome
Probably due to degenerative changes in the inner ear. The patient complains of attacks of tinnitus, giddiness and progressive deafness.

Treatment. (1) Sedatives are of value, especially those with a selective labyrinthine action such as Stemetil. (2) It improves spotaneously, as the deafness increases, but if very severe, then the inner ear is destroyed surgically.

Nose

The nose is divided into two compartments by the nasal septum. From the lateral walls the three tubinates protrude increasing the surface area for warming and humidifying the inhaled air. The air sinuses and the naso lacrymal duct drain into the nose.

RHINITIS
Inflammation of the mucous membrane of the nose.

Acute
Commonly the result of a viral infection and presents as a head cold.

Chronic
May develop as a result of repeated attacks of acute rhinitis, or as a result of exposure to irritants such as industrial gases.

Treatment
Remove the cause if possible.

CHRONIC ALLERGIC RHINITIS
An allergic condition caused by pollen, and dust, especially house dust. The mucous membrane becomes oedematous, blocking the nasal passages and leading to a chronic nasal obstruction with a clear rhinorrhoea and excessive sneezing.

It is helped by nasal decongestants and steroids and, if necessary, cautery.

NASAL POLYPS
Collections of the oedematous mucosa of the turbinates often the result of a long standing allergic rhinitis.

Clinical features
These are similar to chronic allergic rhinitis.

Treatment
Surgical excision.

DEVIATED NASAL SEPTUM
A deviation of the nasal septum can be congenital or post-traumatic. The effect is nasal obstruction and interference with the drainage of the air sinuses.

Treatment
Treatment is by surgical correction.

AIR SINUSES
These are hollow spaces in the facial bones, which are lined with mucous membrane and communicate with the nose.

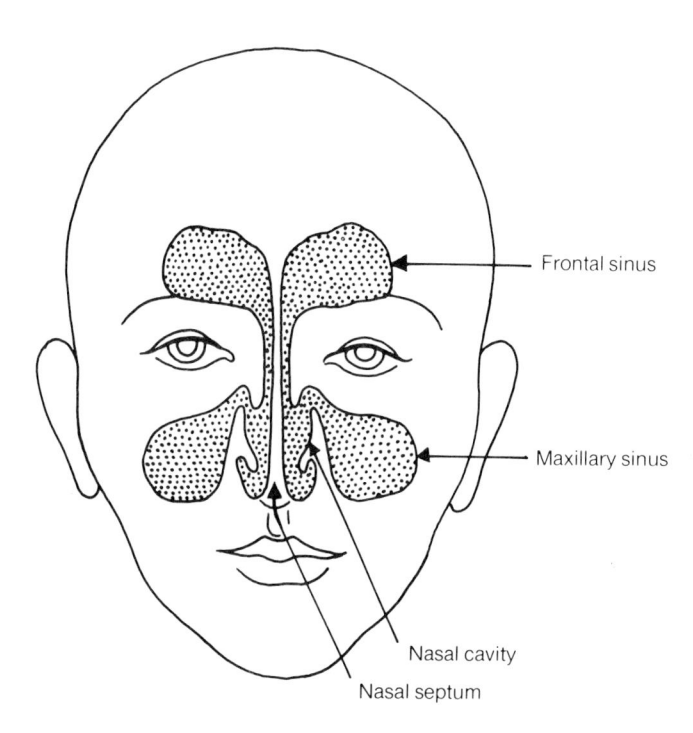

Figure 16.5
Frontal and maxillary sinuses draining into nose

SINUSITIS
Inflammation of the nasal sinuses is often secondary to rhinitis. Frontal sinusitis presents as forehead pain and often headaches. Headaches may also be associated with maxillary sinusitis, as well as cheek pain. Toothache of the upper teeth can be a feature if the roots of the teeth lie in the maxillary sinus.

Treatment
Nasal decongestants are given in order to encourage drainage. It may become chronic and require surgery to allow drainage of the sinuses.

TUMOURS
Carcinoma may develop in the nose or, more likely, in an air sinus.

Clinical features
Progressive blockage of the nose or a sinus with possibly a blood stained nasal discharge.

Treatment
Treatment is mainly by radiotherapy, with surgery for recurrence.

EPISTAXIS
Epistaxis is nasal haemorrhage.

Aetiology
1. *Local.* The vast majority are due to bleeding from the anterior part of the nasal septum (Little's area) and are caused by inflammation from infection, or trauma.
    It can also be caused by nasal or naso pharyngeal tumours.
2. *General.* It can be a feature of a systemic disease such as hypertension or leukaemia.

Treatment
1. Haemorrhage from Little's area usually stop spontaneously, but occasionally cautery of the bleeding area may be necessary.
2. Persistent recurring bleeding may require to be controlled by anterior or posterior nasal packs.

17 Breast

The breast is composed of many *lobules* of glandular tissue interspersed with fat. The lobules are supported by a framework of fibrous tissue grouped together into approximately fifteen *lobes*. The milk from each lobe is gathered by ducts. The ducts unite to form one *lactiferous duct* for each lobe, which opens at the apex of the nipple.

1. *Ovaries.* (a) Oestrogens, which stimulate duct growth in the first half of the menstrual period. (b) Progesterone, which stimulates glandular growth in the second half of the menstrual period.
2. *Placenta* produces oestrogens and progesterone, which continue the preparation of the breast for lactation during pregnancy.
3. *Anterior pituitary* secretes the hormone prolactin, which stimulates milk production after birth.

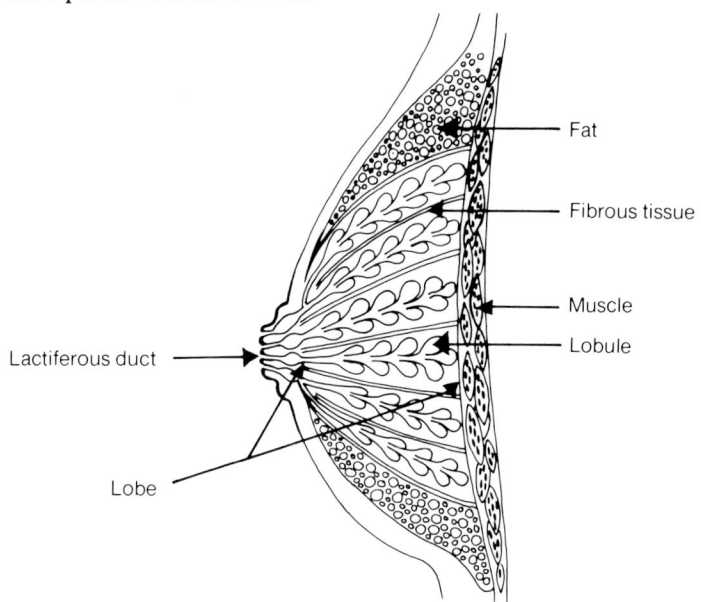

Figure 17.1 Breast

Mastitis

Mastitis is inflammation of the breast.

AETIOLOGY

Hormonal
Develops when the hormone levels are changing.

1. Stimulated by the mother's hormones crossing the placenta (neonatal mastitis).
2. Puberty (affects males and females).

Clinical features
The breast tissue is *swollen* and *tender*. In the infant a drop of milk may be squeezed from the nipple.

Treatment
None is required, for the breast tissue settles when the hormone levels return to normal.

Bacterial
The lactating breast is especially at risk, for the milk is a good culture medium. They are usually Staphylococcal infections.

Clinical features
1. The breast is reddened, swollen and tender (cellulitis).
2. The patient may be pyrexial.

Treatment
1. Antibiotics, e.g. Cloxacillin 2 g/day.
2. Firm bandaging for support.
3. If it does not quickly resolve, then lactation is stopped with stilboestrol 10 mg/day/week.

Breast abscess

Starts as mastitis, subsequently progressing to abscess (p. 10).

Clinical features
1. Initially signs and symptoms of mastitis.
2. There is now a localised fluctant abscess.

Treatment
1. Incision and drainage.
2. Followed by antibiotics, and if still lactating, stilboestrol 10 mg/day/week.

Fibroadenosis

(Chronic mastitis, fibrocystic disease). This condition is probably caused by an imbalance of hormones, which causes over stimulation of the breast tissue.

This results in hyperplasia of cells, causing dilatation of the ducts and glands which go on to form cysts, which are filled with clear brown fluid. There is *no* connection with malignancy.

Clinical features
1. The breasts feel lumpy and are often tender on palpation.
2. Large cysts are felt as smooth swellings.
3. The breasts are often painful, especially before menstruation.

Treatment
1. Reassurance.
2. A good supporting brassiere helps.
3. Biopsy of any swelling which is doubtful.

Tumours

FIBROADENOMA
A benign tumour of fibrous and glandular tissue. Does not become malignant. It is seen in young women as a mobile, painless lump.

Treatment
Local excision.

DUCT PAPILLOMA
A small papilloma developing in a lactiferous duct. It presents as a discharge (often bloody) from the nipple.

Treatment
Excision of a block of breast tissue, containing the duct, for they can become malignant.

CARCINOMA
Arises from the epithelial cells of the ducts, usually in women over forty years old. It occasionally develops in males.

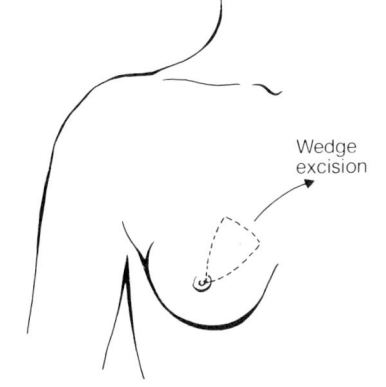

Figure 17.2
Excision of a duct papilloma (removal of a wedge of breast tissue)

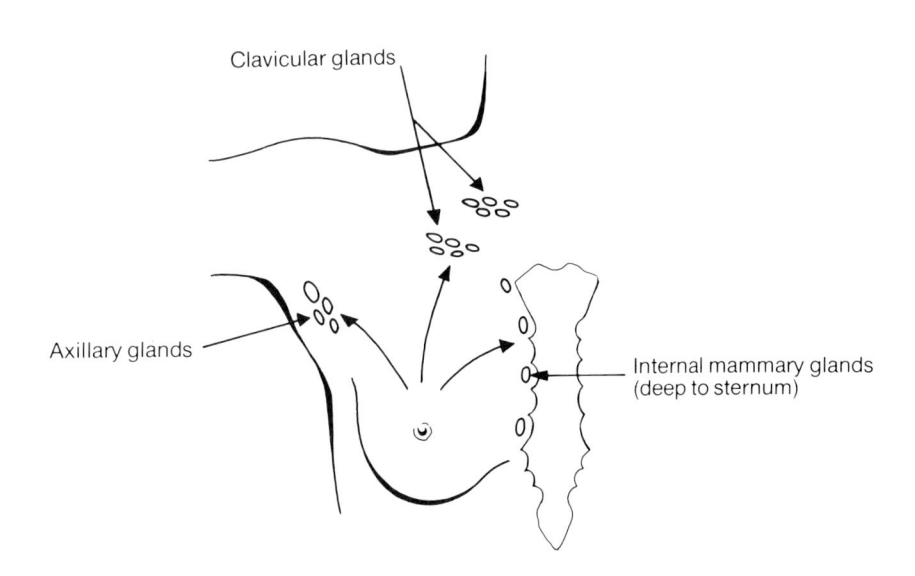

Figure 17.3
Spread of carcinoma

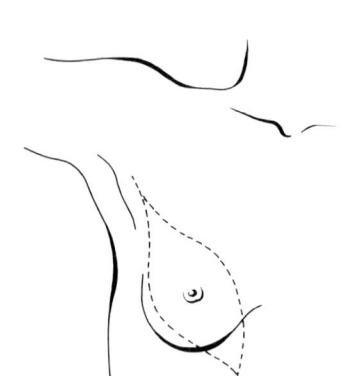

Figure 17.4
Simple mastectomy

Clinical features
1. Presents as a painless, ill-defined lump.
2. May be attached to skin (skin dimpling) and deep structures.
3. May spread to cause enlarged axillary glands.
4. Advanced carcinoma can present as an ulcer.

Spread
1. Local spread leads to skin ulceration.
2. Lymphatic spread is to the lymph glands, especially axillary.
3. Blood spread is usually later and involves the lungs, liver and bones.

Treatment
1. An excision biopsy is carried out and examined immediately under the microscope (frozen section).
2. If malignancy is confirmed the breast is removed—simple mastectomy.
3. Many operations are followed by radiotherapy to the lymph glands, in case the malignancy has spread to them.

Whole body scan
It is now possible to give the patient radioactive phosphorus. This is concentrated in metastases, and the increase in radioactivity in any bone of the body can then be detected by special instruments.

ADVANCED OR RECURRENT CARCINOMA OF BREAST
Some breast carcinomas require oestrogen for cellular division (mitosis) and if deprived they shrink and metastases may recede and even disappear. But it is never a permanent cure and the tumour returns, although it may take years for this to happen.

The oestrogen level can be lowered by:
1. *Oophorectomy* (removal of ovaries).
2. *Anti-oestrogen drugs*, which block the uptake of oestrogen by the tumour—Tamoxiphen 20 mg/day.
3. *Testosterone* (male hormone) reduces the oestrogen effect and thus effects response in some cases.
4. *Adrenalectomy.* Some oestrogens also are produced in the adrenals and excision of these glands (after oophorectomy) may give a second favourable response. As all the adrenal hormones are lost: patients must take daily *cortisone* for it is essential for life.
5. *Hypophysectomy.* The anterior pituitary (hormone ACTH) stimulates adrenal secretions (p. 190). Removing the anterior pituitary reduces the adrenal hormones and has a similar effect to adrenalectomy.

The first and second may be used at the initial treatment, but the third and fourth and fifth are reserved for recurrence.

18 Thorax

The thoracic viscera are protected by the semi-rigid cage formed by the ribs. The ribs articulate posteriorly with the vertebrae and anteriorly with the sternum through the costal cartilages. These articulations allow the movement necessary for respiration. But the elevation of the rib cage on inspiration is dependent on the rigidity of the ribs which is lost with multiple fractures (p. 79). The diaphragm closes the thorax inferiorly from the abdomen. *The pleura* a slippery membrane, forms a closed sac or cavity, which lines and is attached to the inside of the chest wall and diaphragm (parietal pleura) and is then reflected at the lung hilum on to the surface of the lung (visceral pleura). There is a little fluid in the sac for lubrication.

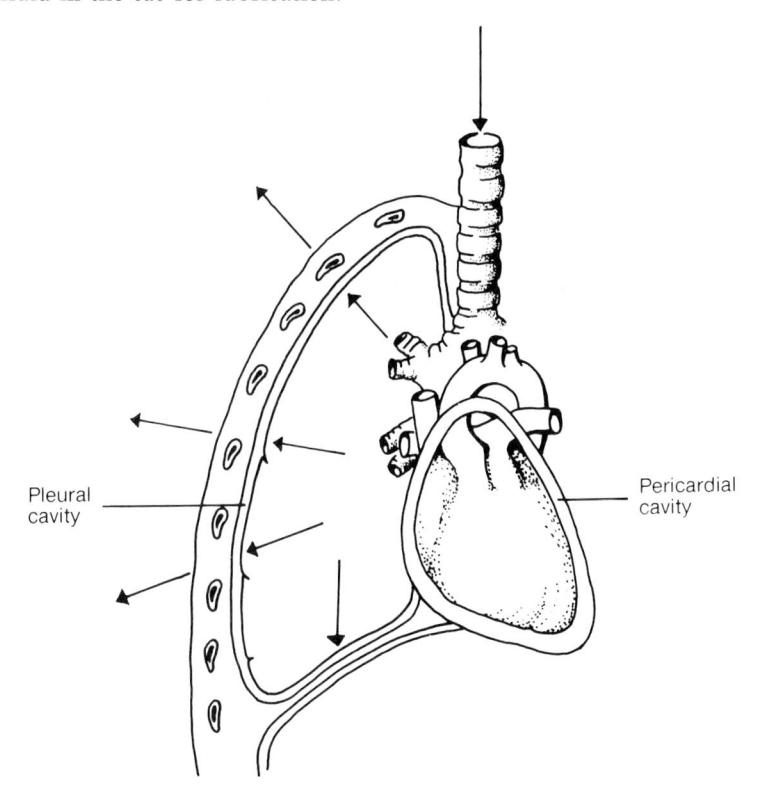

Figure 18.1
Thorax – showing action of inspiration

The heart is enclosed in a similar way: *the pericardium* forms a closed sac with a free parietal layer, reflected at the great vessels on to the surface of the heart (visceral pericardium).

Respiration

The pressure in the chest is normally below atmospheric pressure. This negative pressure or suction keeps the lung expanded against the chest wall.

On inspiration, air is pulled through the trachea and bronchi to the lungs by an increase in thoracic volume.

The thoracic volume is increased by:
1. Elevation of the ribs.
2. Contraction and lowering of the diaphragm.

Chest injuries

Chest injuries may be:
1. *Open* injuries.
2. *Closed* injuries which may be
   a. *penetrating* injury.
   b. *crushing* injury (e.g. fractured ribs, crushed chest).

OPEN INJURY

A large lacerated wound, where there may be loss of part of the chest wall. The pleura is open and the lung collapsed. Air is sucked in through the wound on inspiration, making respiration very difficult.

Clinical features
1. A large open wound, which may 'suck' with inspiration and 'blow' on expiration.
2. A very shocked and probably cyanotic patient struggling to breathe.

Treatment
1. Immediate closure of defect by a pad, adhesive dressing, or even a hand greatly assists respiration.
2. Emergency surgery to clean the wound, and close the defect.
3. Water-sealed drainage of the pleural cavity to expand the lung.

Water-sealed drain. This is a large bottle with several inches of sterile water in it, which stands on the floor. The tube from the chest drain goes one inch below the water level. Air can escape from the chest by bubbling out through the water, but the water, which prevents air entering on inspiration, is too heavy to be sucked up the tube. All cases after chest surgery have a water sealed drain.

CLOSED INJURY

Penetrating (e.g. stab or bullet wound)
The wound penetrates the chest wall and the lung. But the wounds are quickly sealed by the elasticity of the tissues and by clot. The chest wall function remains normal.

Clinical features
These depend on the internal structures damaged and can vary from virtually nil, through pneumothorax, haemothorax (air or blood in the pleural cavity) to instant death, if the heart or great vessels are involved.

Treatment
1. Careful monitoring in order that complications are recognised early.
2. Cleansing and suturing of wounds.

Crushing injury
The injury is a blow or crushing, which fractures the ribs, but does not penetrate the chest wall. The degree of injury ranges from a single fractured rib to a crushed chest with multiple fractures. Any case may have internal damage, especially those with multiple fractures.

Fractured rib
Usually caused by a blow or by being crushed; but a violent cough may do it.

Clinical features
1. There is a sharp pain and tenderness at the fracture site, especially on respiration.
2. There may be crepitus (grating of the bone ends).

Treatment
1. Analgesics—to combat the pain which inhibits the patient coughing and leads to retention of secretions.
2. Strapping to the chest wall if the pain is severe.
   The fracture heals in about three weeks.

Crushed chest
Caused by severe trauma often in a car crash. There is resultant injury to (1) the chest wall (2) the internal structures.

Injury to the chest wall
Multiple fractured ribs make respiration difficult. There may be *paradoxical respiration* where the fractures have created a *loose segment* of chest wall which, being unsupported, is *sucked in on inspiration and blown out on expiration*. In severe cases the whole side of the chest may be loose (flail chest) and respiration is gravely embarrassed.

Clinical features are as follows:
1. Breathing is heaving and rapid as the patient fights to get oxygen.
2. Cyanosis may be marked in severe cases.
3. Paradoxical respiration may be present.
4. There is often severe shock.
5. Haemoptysis may be present from injury to the lung.

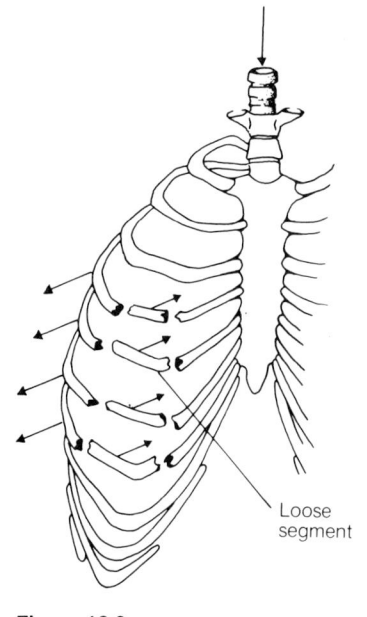

Figure 18.2
Paradoxical respiration (inspiration)

Treatment. Severe cases require immediate positive pressure respiration using initially an anaesthetic endo tracheal tube, which is replaced later by a tracheostomy tube (p. 66). The tube is connected to a ventilator which automatically inflates and deflates the lungs until the chest wall has healed sufficiently and regained its rigidity to allow the patient to manage without help. The normal respiratory impulses are inhibited by drugs to prevent conflict with the machine.

Biochemical measurements are vital for this treatment. Starting on admission, frequent checks on the oxygen and carbon dioxide levels in the blood are made. The depth and speed of respiration by the machine are regulated to keep these blood levels normal. Frequent electrolyte and Ph checks are also required (p. 29).

Less severe cases respond to adequate analgesia, intensive physiotherapy and antibiotics, if the sputum becomes infected.

Injury to internal structures
The visceral pleura and lung may be pierced by a rib causing a pneumothorax or a haemothorax. These will further embarrass respiration and are serious complications.

Treatment. An immediate chest drain, which is protected by an underwater seal (p. 78) no replacement of blood loss.

SURGICAL EMPHYSEMA
Damage to the lung and pleura by a sharp fractured rib end can allow the escape of air into the pleural cavity and the tissue of the chest wall (surgical emphysema). It then spreads to the neck, face and abdomen.

Clinical features
Gross puffiness of the tissues, which 'crackle' on palpation (crepitation).

Treatment
None is required for it is reabsorbed when the leak in the lung has healed. Treatment will usually be required for the accompanying pneumothorax.

VASCULAR INJURY
Injury to the pericardium can fill the closed sac with blood, making it increasingly difficult for the heart to expand and fill with returning venous blood (cardiac tamponade). The neck veins become congested and the pulse rapid and feeble, leading eventually to death as the heart is compressed.

Treatment
Is immediate tapping of the pericardial sac with a needle. The heart and great vessels may also be damaged and they may require surgical repair.

PNEUMOTHORAX
Air in the pleural cavity.

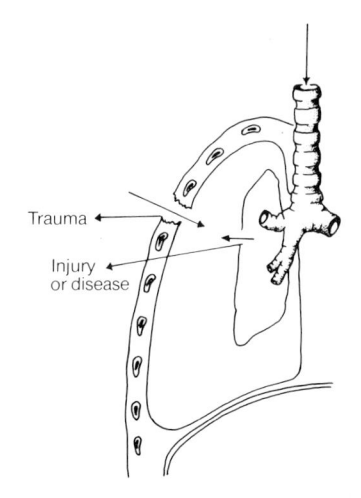

Figure 18.3 Pneumothorax

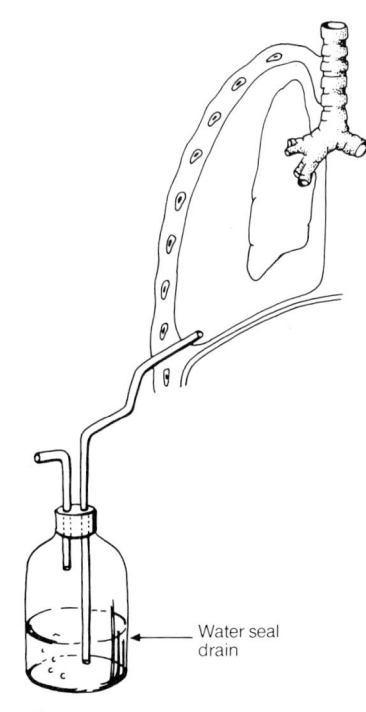

Figure 18.4 Pneumothorax with chest drain

Aetiology

Traumatic
1. Through the chest wall (open pneumothorax) (p. 78).
2. From a punctured lung.
3. Post-operative after surgery of the lung.

Spontaneous
Diseases of the lung may weaken the visceral pleura, which ruptures and the air passages then open into the pleural cavity, e.g. tuberculosis, emphysema.

Pathology
As the air enters the lung collapses and the hole in the lung becomes sealed. In some cases, air continues to enter and, as it cannot escape, the volume of the pneumothorax increases and pushes the mediastinum over, compressing the other lung (tension pneumothorax).

Clinical features
1. Sudden chest pain with breathlessness.
2. In tension pneumothorax the breathlessness increases and cyanosis develops.
3. If unrelieved, asphyxia and death follow.

Treatment
1. If small it should be left to be reabsorbed.
2. If large, drain chest with one-way valve or under-water sealed drain.

Tension pneumothorax is an *emergency*.

HAEMOTHORAX
Blood in the pleural cavity.

Aetiology
1. Trauma
   a. From chest wall.
   b. Internal organs.
   c. Post operative.
2. Medical
   a. Complications of spontaneous pneumothorax.
   b. Dissecting aneurysm of the aorta.
   c. Malignant disease.

Clinical features
1. Similar to pleural effusion (p. 82) but chest pain is more pronounced.
2. Patient may be shocked if it occurs suddenly.

Treatment
1. Traumatic cases require a chest drain.

2. Non-traumatic cases are aspirated and investigated to find the cause.
3. Blood transfusion if the patient is shocked.

PLEURAL EFFUSION
Excess fluid in the pleural cavity.

Aetiology (See Fig. 18.5)
1. Infection
   a. From the lung, e.g. pneumonia, tuberculosis.
   b. From the chest wall, e.g. infected wound.
   c. Spread from the abdomen, e.g. subphrenic abscess.
2. Malignant Disease – primary carcinoma of bronchus (A).
3. Vascular Cause – Pulmonary embolus (B).

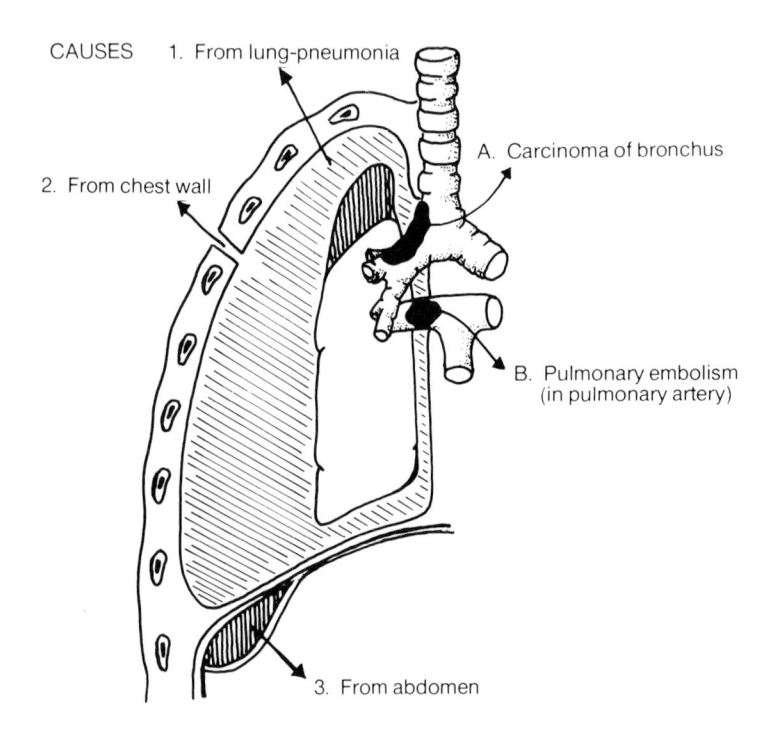

Figure 18.5
Pleural effusion

Clinical features
1. Dyspnoea on exertion, or at rest if it is large.
2. Slight pain in the chest on breathing.
3. Less chest movement on that side.
4. May be pyrexia.

Treatment
1. Aspiration. This also allows fluid to be investigated for bacteria and malignant cells.
2. Treatment of the cause, i.e. antibiotics, etc.

If it has an infective cause, it can become empyema thoracis.

EMPYEMA THORACIS

Pus in the pleural cavity may follow an infective effusion and become sealed off as an abscess. In addition it can be a post-operative complication.

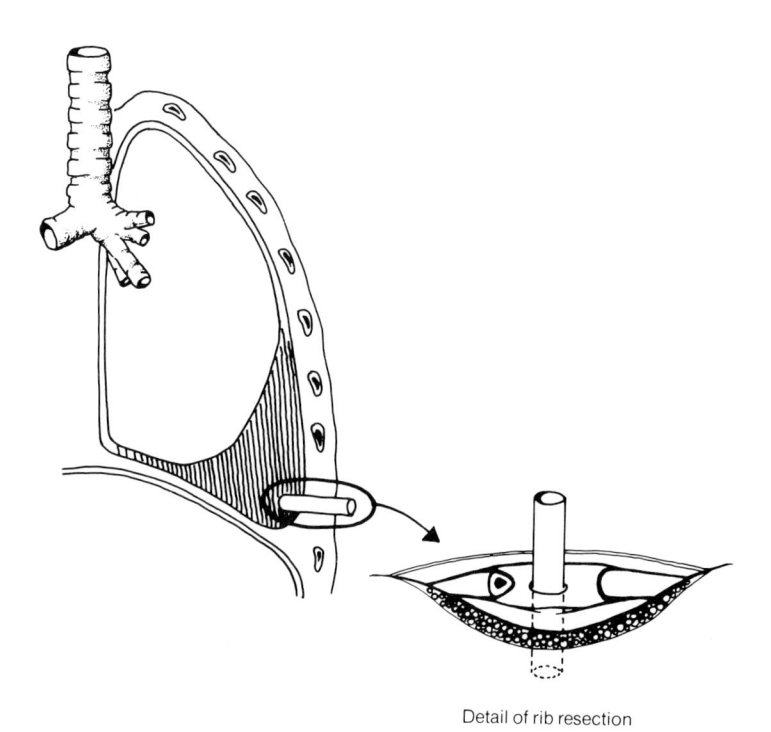

Figure 18.6
Drainage of empyema by rib resection

Detail of rib resection

Treatment
1. Antibiotics.
2. Repeated aspirations.
3. May require surgery (decortication) to re-expand the lung and continuous drainage by removal of part of a rib for some weeks to allow the cavity to become obliterated.

Decortication is excision of the granulation and scar tissue.

LUNG ABSCESS

They are now rare (excluding those caused by malignancy). Most arise as a complication of pneumonia, especially staphylococcal pneumonia. They respond to antibiotics and postural drainage (physiotherapy).

Tumours

BENIGN

Benign tumours of the lung are rare. They are usually removed because it is impossible to distinguish them from carcinomas.

MALIGNANT

1. Primary. Carcinoma of bronchus is now the commonest cancer affecting man.
2. Secondary. Malignancy is also very common arising mainly from breast, kidneys, testes, etc.

Carcinoma of bronchus

Main aetiological factor in carcinoma of bronchus is smoking. It arises usually from the mucous membrane of the larger bronchi. It spreads to the mediastinal lymph nodes and also by the blood to the liver, brain and skeleton.

Clinical features
1. A cough with blood stained sputum caused by irritation.
2. It may obstruct the bronchus causing distal lung collapse, (atelectasis) which is often followed by infection.
3. Spread to the pleura causes pleural effusion.
4. Enlarged malignant glands in the mediastinum can block by compression, e.g.
    a. Vena cava—plethoric face—from venous congestion.
    b. Oesophagus—dysphagia.
    c. Laryngeal nerve paralysis by direct invasion (p. 66). There is also hoarseness.
5. It may present first with a distant metastases, e.g. epileptic fits from a cerebral metastases.

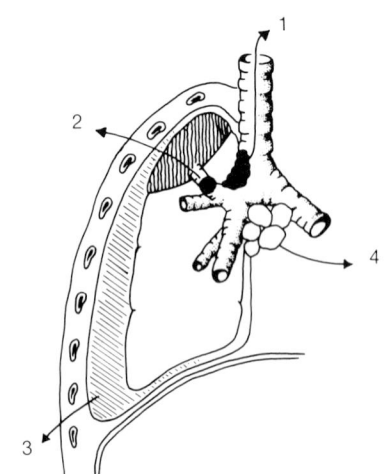

Figure 18.7
Carcinoma of bronchus (clinical features)
1. Cough and blood stained sputum
2. Obstructed bronchus—lung collapse and infection
3. Pleural effusion
4. Enlarged mediastinal glands

Treatment
1. Lung resection (pneumonectomy or lobectomy) for a possible cure. Most are inoperable when first seen.
2. Radiotherapy or cytotoxics for palliation.

Congenital heart and aortic disease

HEART

Septal defects
These are congenital failures of the wall between the atria or between the ventricles to complete their development leaving 'gaps' or defects between the chambers. This results in blood shunting from the left (high pressure) side of the heart to the right (low pressure) and so greatly increasing the pulmonary circulation at the expense of the systemic circulation, which is reduced. The shunt greatly increases the work load of the right side of the heart and may cause eventually its failure. A similar situation exists in patent ductus arteriosis—see below, (p. 85).

Treatment
Surgical closure.

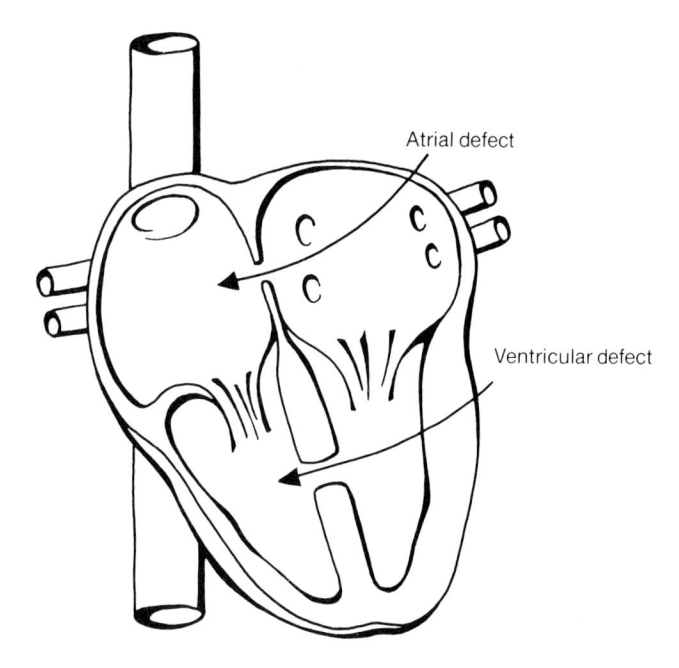

Figure 18.8
Septal defects

Valvular defects
The valves of the heart may be involved by congenital or acquired disease and become stenosed (narrowed) or incompetent (not closed properly). Both conditions cause the heart to work harder and eventually cause cardiac failure.

Treatment
It is possible to replace each of the heart valves with an artificial one.

PATENT DUCTUS ARTERIOSIS
Before birth, as the lungs are not required, most of the blood by-passes them through a duct from the pulmonary artery to the aorta. This should close automatically at birth, but occasionally remains open and blood from the aorta enters the pulmonary circulation. The pulmonary circulatory volume is consequently much larger and the work of the heart is greatly increased by this and by trying to maintain the systemic circulation despite the aortic 'leak'. Eventually the heart may fail.

Treatment
Surgical ligation of the duct.

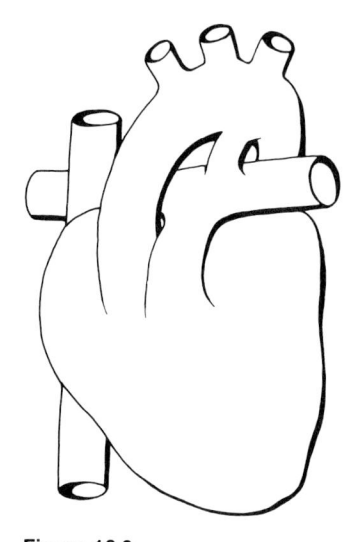

Figure 18.9
Patent ductus arteriosus

COARCTATION OF THE AORTA
A congenital narrowing of the aorta causing a very high blood pressure in the head and arms of young people and a low blood pressure in the rest of the body.

Treatment
Surgical excision and anastomosis of proximal and distal aorta.

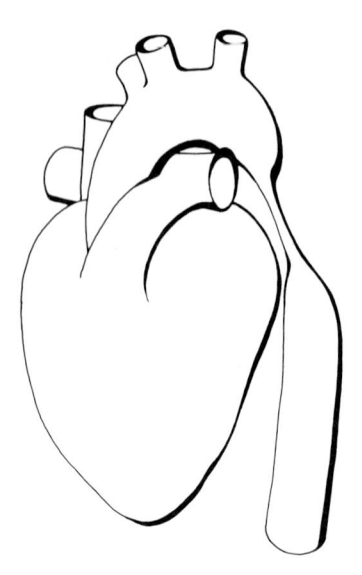

Figure 18.10
Co-arctation of aorta

ACQUIRED HEART DISASE

Mitral stenosis
The result of rheumatic heart disease, the valve is thickened by the cusps becoming stuck together and its orifice narrowed. This causes the blood to be dammed back in the lungs and increases the work of the right ventricle as it pushes the blood through the lungs. If the narrowing is severe enough, heart failure may develop.

Treatment
Surgically split the cusps open (mitral valvotomy). Frequently the valve may require to be replaced (but this is a much more major operation).

Coronary heart disease
As a result of arteriosclerosis (p. 37). If the narrowing of the artery is localised it is now possible to by-pass it with a vein graft using a portion of vein removed from the leg.

Coronary artery by-pass graft (CABG) is the most frequently performed heart operation at the present time.

Heart lung machine

A machine which can maintain the *oxygenation* and *circulation* of the blood to the vital centres, especially the brain and the kidneys. Using this machine *the heart can be isolated from the circulation* and opened to allow surgery inside the chambers, e.g. valve replacement. At the start of the operation and after giving heparin to prevent the blood clotting in the machine, cannulae are placed in both vena cavae and the venous blood diverted to the machine. After oxygenation and removal of carbon dioxide it is pumped into the aorta through a further cannula. After surgery, the cannulae are removed, the incisions in the great vessels sutured and the heparin neutralised.

19 Oesophagus

A muscular tube lined by squamous epithelium. It is continuous with the pharynx in the neck, then passes through the posterior mediastinum of the thorax to end in the abdomen at the cardia of the stomach. The bolus of food from the pharynx is carried by peristalsis to the stomach. The cardiac sphincter at the lower end of the oesophagus which is normally closed to stop regurgitation opens and allows the bolus to enter the stomach.

Investigations

BARIUM SWALLOW
Barium is swallowed and its passage watched and filmed with X-rays. Irregularities of the mucous membrane and alteration in peristalsis can be seen.

OESOPHAGOSCOPE
An instrument which is passed down the oesophagus giving a direct view of the mucous membrane. Through it a biopsy can be taken.

PRESSURE STUDIES
Recently tiny pressure gauges attached to modified naso gastric tubes have been used to investigate oesophageal disorders of peristalsis by measuring the intra luminal pressures.

Congenital atresia of the oesophagus

There is a failure of a segment of the oesophagus to develop and the proximal and distal portions may end in blind pouches. Most cases, however, have an associated tracheo-oesophageal fistula where one or both portions open into the trachea.

This results in all food and saliva being regurgitated, or it enters the trachea.

Clinical features
1. Saliva may run from the new-born child's mouth (due to the blockage).
2. From the first, the child regurgitates its feeds.
3. Especially when feeding the child coughs and becomes cyanosed.

Treatment
1. All feeding by mouth is stopped.

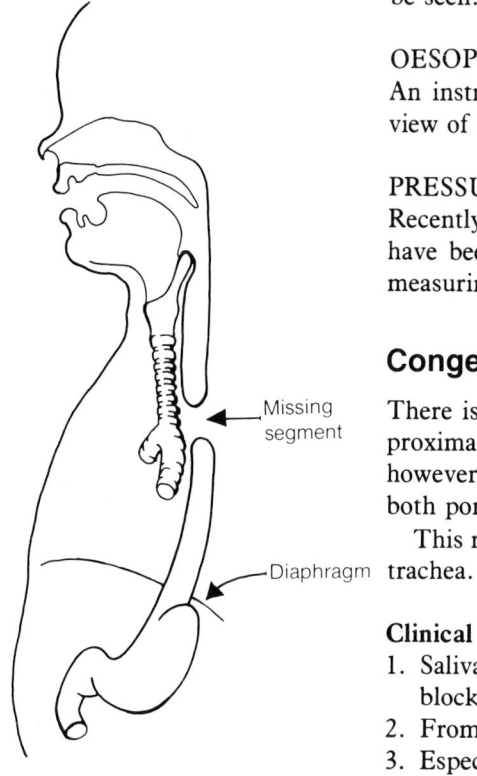

Figure 19.1
Oesophagus—atresia of the oesophagus

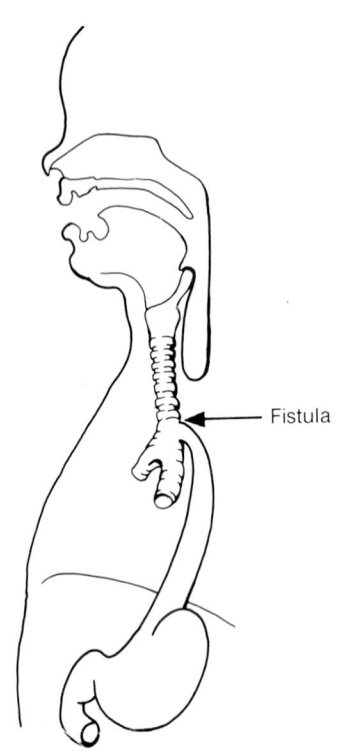

Figure 19.2
Oesophagus—atresia with trachea oesophageal fistula

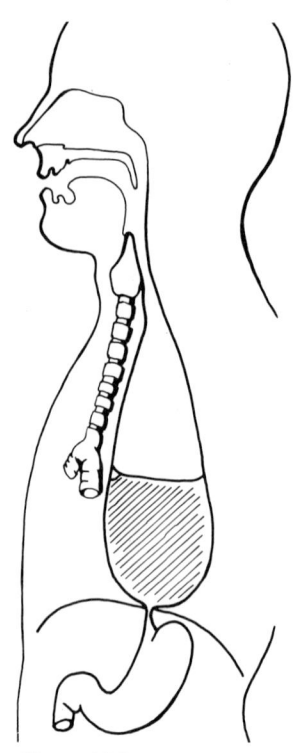

Figure 19.3
Achalasia of oesophagus

2. Surgical repair of the fistula and establishment of continuity of the oesophagus is performed usually by anastomosis of the two ends.

Plummer-Vinson syndrome

Spasm of the muscle at the *upper* end of oesophagus with gradual fibrous tissue replacement of the muscle and permanent narrowing. Associated with long-standing iron deficiency *anaemia*.

Clinical features
1. Slowly progressive dysphagia (difficulty in swallowing).
2. Signs of long-standing anaemia.

Treatment
1. Gentle dilatation (bouginage) which is repeated when necessary.
2. Correction of anaemia.

Achalasia (cardiospasm)

Spasm of the lower circular muscle fibres of the oesophagus, which will not relax to allow the bolus of food to pass (i.e. disordered peristalsis). It is a progressive condition with gradual dilatation of the proximal oesophagus to accommodate the contents. Eventually nothing enters the stomach. The cause is unknown.

Clinical features
1. Progressive dysphagia over a long period.
2. Regurgitation of food (pseudo-vomiting).
3. Loss of weight and ill health.

Treatment
1. Regular dilatation (bouginage) stretches the spastic muscles and keeps the oesophageal lumen open.
2. *Surgery.* Division of the spastic circular muscle fibres at the constriction (Heller's operation), permanently cures the condition.

Hiatus hernia

The proximal portion of the stomach with the abdominal oesophagus with the cardiac sphincter pass (herniate) through the oesophageal hiatus into the thorax (sliding), or part of the fundus of the stomach only may pass through to lie beside the oesophagus (para-oesophageal).

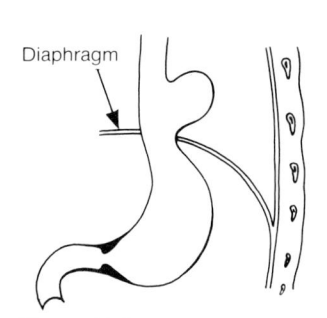

Figure 19.4 Sliding hiatus hernia

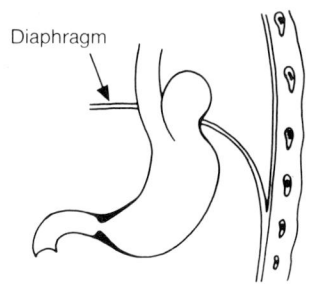

Figure 19.5 Para-oesophageal hiatus hernia

Aetiology
1. Increased abdominal pressure force them through, e.g. obesity or tight corsets, or both.
2. Weakness of diaphragmatic muscles with age.

Result
The cardiac sphincter may become incompetent and so allow the reflux of gastric juice, which attacks the oesophagus causing *oesophagitis* and eventually ulceration (peptic ulceration) (p. 104).

Clinical features
1. There may be none if there is no regurgitation.
2. *Heartburn* (searing sensation behind sternum), which may be triggered off by bending or lying down (as gastric juice runs up the oesophagus).

Treatment

1. *Oesophagitis*
   a. Antacids to reduce the acid in the gastric juice, e.g. magnesium trisilicate, aluminium hydroxide or cimethidine (p. 105).
   b. Reduce weight by diet (reducing the abdominal pressure).
   c. Remove constrictive clothing for the same reason.
   d. Avoid bending to stop gastric juice regurgitation.
   e. Sleep with head of bed raised nine inches for the same reason.

Often these measures are enough, but if not surgical repair is necessary.

2. *Surgical repair*
   The oesophagus and stomach are returned to the abdomen and the hernia repaired by narrowing the excessive gap in the oesophageal hiatus with sutures.

Complications
Chronic *oesophagitis*, which results in peptic *ulceration* and in turn the complications of
1. Bleeding
2. Stricture (stenosis)

Carcinoma of the oesophagus

Commonest in elderly men. It is a squamous cell carcinoma, which grows round the oesophageal wall and so blocking the lumen. It grows fairly slowly and spreads to the nearest lymph glands in the neck, chest or abdomen. Tumours of the distal oesophagus are often adenocarcinomas from glandular tissue.

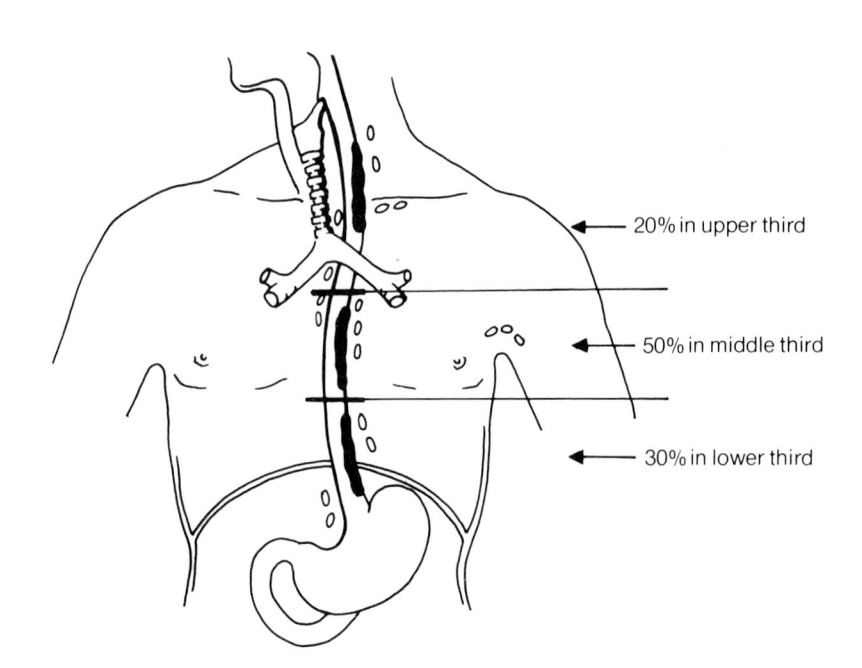

Figure 19.6
Incidence of carcinoma of oesophagus

- 20% in upper third
- 50% in middle third
- 30% in lower third

Clinical features
1. Progressive dysphagia firstly to solids, then liquids and eventually a complete blockage.
2. Regurgitation of food caused by the progressive blockage.
3. Loss of weight.
4. Anaemia.

Treatment
This may be *curative* or *palliative* depending on the site and the size of the tumour.

Upper third—radiotherapy (curative or palliative)
Surgery is too hazardous.

Middle third—surgery
After removal of the whole distal portion of the oesophagus down to the stomach, the cardia is closed. The stomach, being very mobile, is then brought up into the chest as a tube and the fundus is anastomosed to the proximal oesophagus.

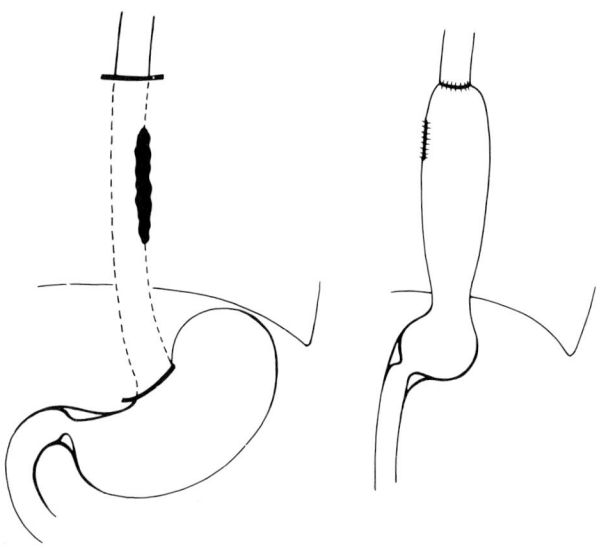

Figure 19.7
Surgery of middle third

Oesophago—gastric anastomosis

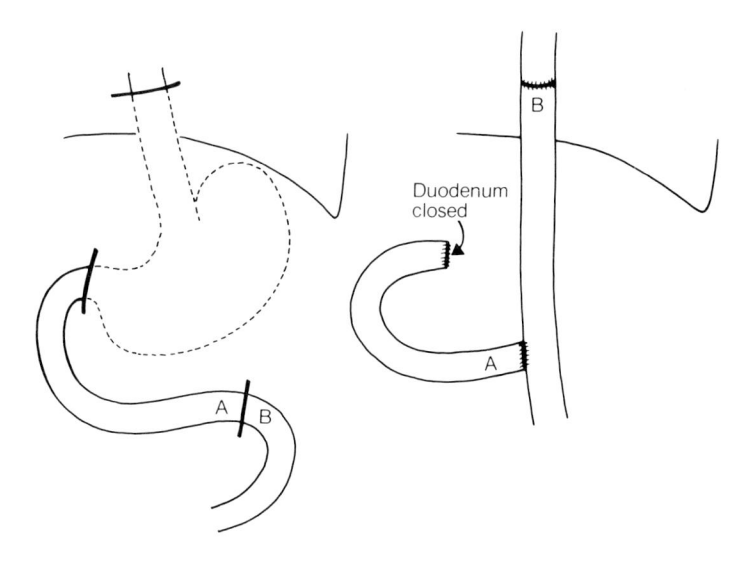

Figure 19.8
Surgery of lower third—removal of oesophagus and stomach

Oesophago—jejunal anastomosis

Radiotherapy
Mainly used for palliation.

Lower third—surgery
The lower end of the oesophagus and the stomach are removed and the proximal oesophagus joined to the small bowel.

Radiotherapy is used for palliation to squamous carcinomas, but adenocarcinomas are resistant to radiotherapy.

Celestin tube
The tube is used for palliation only where the inoperable tumour is obstructing the lumen. At operation, a plastic, funnel-shaped tube is guided through the obstructed lumen. The upper funnel lies above the tumour and the distal end opens into the stomach. This allows the patient to eat and drink normally.

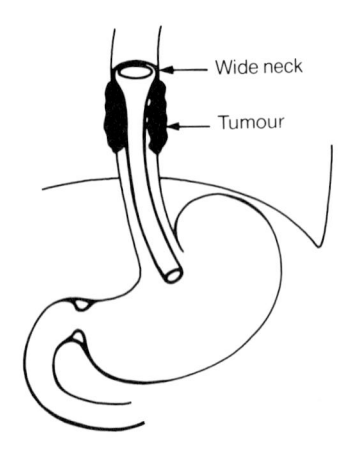

Figure 19.9
Celestin tube *in situ*

20 Peritoneum

The peritoneum is a layer of cells lining the abdominal and pelvic cavities. Developing organs bulge into and *fill* the cavity but only by becoming covered by the peritoneal layer. Only a potential space is left—the peritoneal cavity—which contains a little fluid to allow movement between organs. In the female, the fallopian tubes open into the cavity.

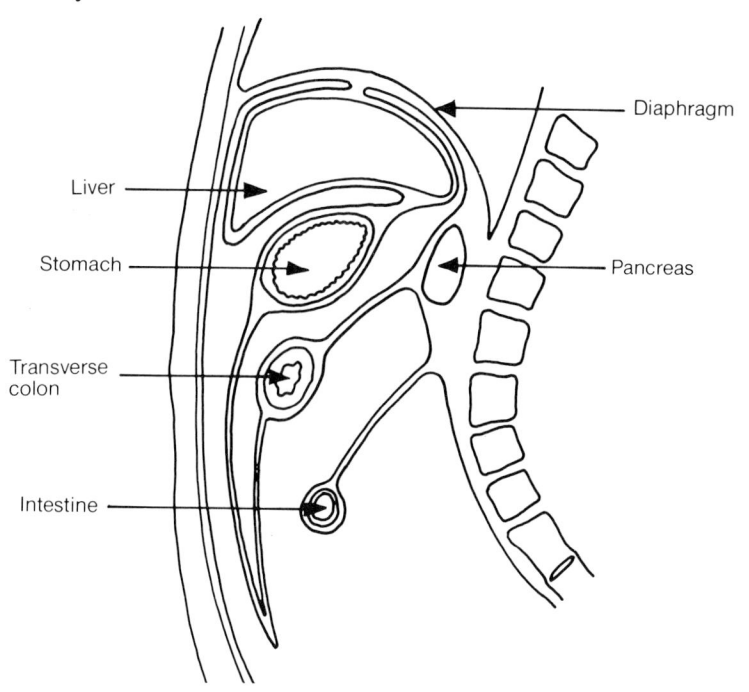

Figure 20.1
Peritoneum

Acute peritonitis

The peritoneum reacts to injury with inflammation (p. 9) and an increase in peritoneal fluid.

Aetiology
1. Infection
   a. Spread from organs—appendix.
   b. From wounds—of abdominal wall or organs.
   c. Result of surgery.
   d. From the fallopian tubes.
2. Chemical, e.g. gastric juice (perforation, p. 107).

INFECTIVE PERITONITIS

Infective peritonitis starts as a local peritonitis and causes a peritoneal reaction.

Peritoneal reaction
1. Inflammation of the peritoneal layer (p. 9), which causes
2. Outpouring of peritoneal fluid, which dilutes the bacterial toxins and contains
    a. Fibrinogen which changes to solid fibrin and is a barrier limiting the spread of the infection.
    b. White blood cells.
    c. Antibodies.
3. Paralytic ileus. Peristalsis ceases in the inflamed bowel, so stopping the spread of the bacteria by the moving intestines (see below). The paralysis may be local or general.

Clinical features

Local peritonitis
1. Features of the causative disease, e.g. appendicitis.
2. Pain, tenderness over the site (local inflammation).
3. Local increased muscle rigidity (nerves stimulated by inflammation).
4. Pyrexia and tachycardia (systemic response).

Treatment
1. Remove the cause if possible, e.g. appendicetomy.
2. Antibiotics, if necessary.

N.B. *Local peritonitis* may spread to be a *general peritonitis*.

Spread depends on:
1. The virulence of the bacteria and
2. The numbers of bacteria present (p. 9).

Prevention of spread depends on the general body resistance and the local peritoneal reaction.

GENERAL PERITONITIS

Clinical features
1. Silent abdomen (paralytic ileus—no bowel sounds).
2. Abdominal distension (result of paralytic ileus).
3. Patient is very ill—marked pyrexia and tachycardia.
4. Patient may be dehydrated and shocked.

Treatment
1. Naso-gastric suction and intravenous drip.
2. Antibiotics.

3. Remove cause if possible.
4. Peritoneal toilet.

Peritoneal toilet
When the peritoneal cavity is opened and the cause removed, as much as possible of the purulent fluid is sucked out. Solutions of an antiseptic (Noxyflex) or an antibiotic (tetracycline, cephalosporin) are sometimes placed in the cavity if the cause is bacterial. On abdominal closure, the peritoneal cavity may be drained to allow the escape of any residual fluid.

Complications
1. Abscess—both local and general peritonitis may lead to abscess formation (p. 10). These will require drainage. They are often very large (500 to 1000 ml) and cause marked systemic responses.
2. Paralytic ileus.

Peritoneal abscess

Clinical features
1. Fluctuating temperature and pulse.
2. Shivering attacks followed by sweating (rigors).
3. Tenderness over site (local inflammation).
4. Leucocytosis.

SUBPHRENIC ABSCESS
Lies below diaphragm, but above the liver.

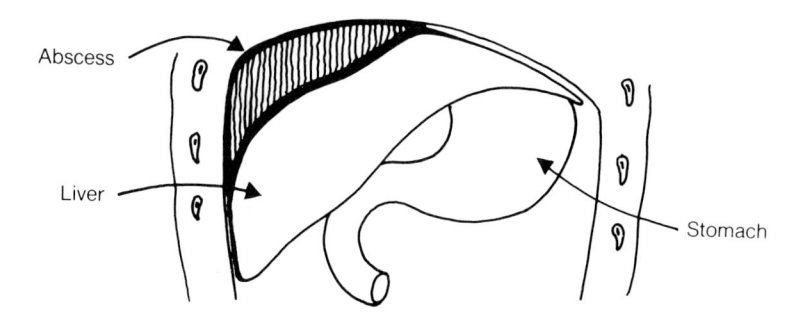

Figure 20.2
Subphrenic abscess

Clinical features
As for abscess, with tenderness and swelling below the ribs.

PELVIC ABSCESS
Lies in the pelvis in front of the rectum and behind the uterus and bladder.

Clinical features
As for abscess, with:
1. Diarrhoea.

2. Bulging abscess felt on rectal examination.
3. It may rupture spontaneously, producing pus in the bedpan.

A pelvic abscess is usually opened and drained through the rectal or vaginal wall.

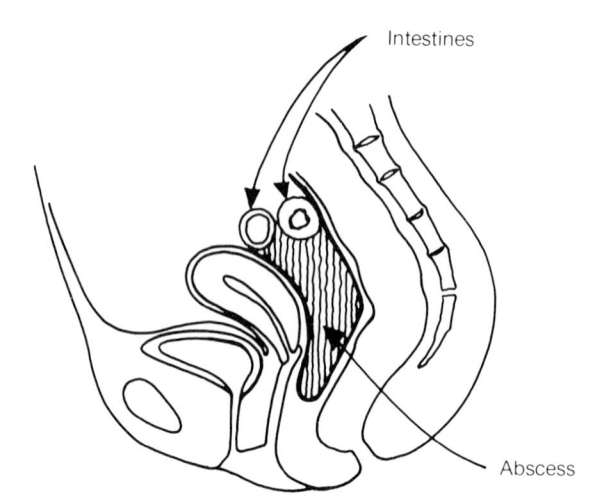

Figure 20.3 Pelvic abscess

Paralytic ileus

Although beneficial in hindering spread of infection, it causes the bowel to distend with gas and fluid (causing dehydration). It is caused by bacterial toxins acting on nerves in bowel wall (see p. 114).

Clinical features
1. Silent abdomen, which is uncomfortable but not painful.
2. Distension due to dilatation of the intestines.
3. Gas and fluid levels on X-ray.
4. Patient may be dehydrated and even shocked.

Treatment
1. Nasogastric tube and suction—to reduce the distension.
2. Intravenous drip to replace fluid lost in bowel or aspirated.
3. Treatment of the cause, e.g. peritonitis.

Adhesions

The end result of the peritoneal exudate (fibrin) forms fibrous bands and plaques joining bowel to itself and other peritoneal surfaces. They can lead to obstruction of the bowel if it should become twisted round these bands.

Chronic peritonitis

Rare now, but was due to tuberculosis causing peritoneal thickening and ascites.

Clinical features
Usually in children or adolescents who present with distended abdomens in association with progressive loss of health and vitality.

Treatment
Anti-tuberculous drugs.

Faecal peritonitis

A particular type of general peritonitis caused by a perforation in the large bowel allowing faeces to enter the peritoneal cavity. It is very serious and has a very high mortality (ulcerative colitis, p. 122, diverticulitis, p. 120).

21 Hernia

A hernia is an escape of the contents of a body cavity—usually the abdomen—through a gap in the surrounding wall.

Description

Abdominal hernias usually consist of a *sac* of peritoneum and the escaped tissues which are usually (not invariably) in the sac and if so are then called the *contents* (e.g. bowel, omentum, etc.). The sac has a mouth, neck, body and fundus. Hernias are of three main types:

Reducible. The escaped tissues return easily to the abdomen.

Irreducible. The escaped tissues cannot easily return to the abdomen because of adhesions to the sac.

Strangulated. The neck of the sac, acts as a tourniquet, blocking the blood flow. The lumen of the bowel is blocked and the bowel itself will become gangrenous in a few hours.

Clinical features of strangulation
1. Pain and tenderness over an irreducible hernia.
2. Signs of intestinal obstruction (p. 114).

Treatment
1. Treatment by gastric suction and intravenous fluid of the obstruction.
2. Emergency operation to relieve the bowel and the obstruction. If it is gangrenous it is resected.
3. Repair of the hernia.

Inguinal hernia

Herniation through the inguinal canal alongside the spermatic cord or round ligament of uterus. It may start at the internal inguinal ring (indirect) or push through a weakened posterior wall of the inguinal canal (direct). It may be present at birth (p. 204).

Clinical features
1. A swelling in inguinal region, above the inguinal ligament, which reduces on lying down.
2. In the male, it may fill the scrotum.

Figure 21.1 Hernia

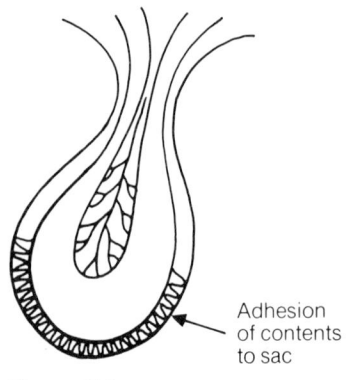

Figure 21.2 Irreducible hernia

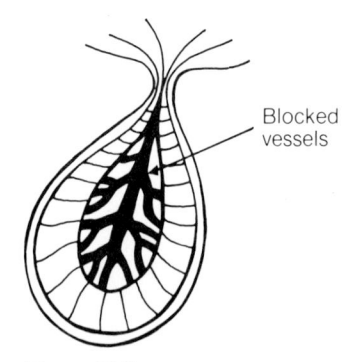

Figure 21.3 Strangulated hernia

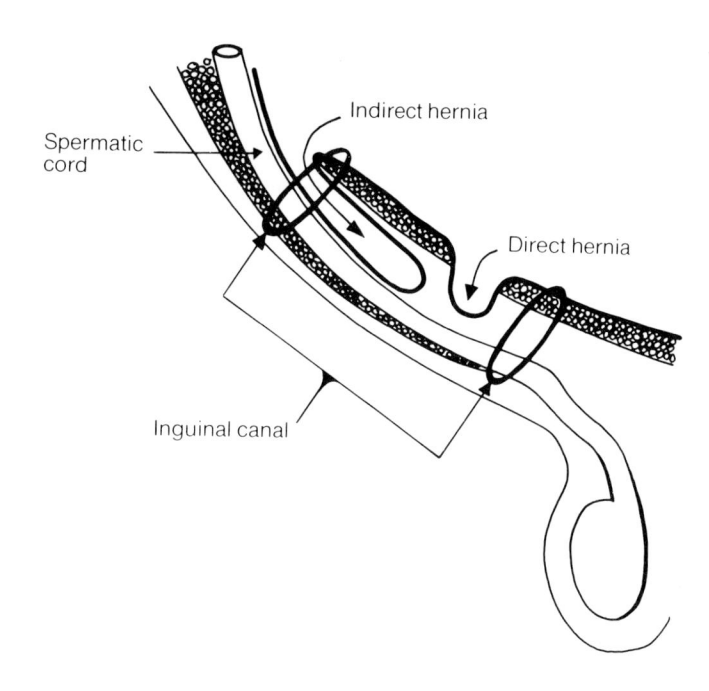

Figure 21.4
Inguinal hernias

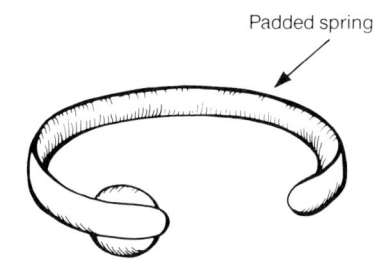

Figure 21.5
Hernia – truss

Treatment

Truss
There are several different types, but they are reserved for the very old or infirm—one type consists of a strong spring and pad which when placed on the neck of the sac keeps it closed by pressure after the contents have been reduced.

Surgery
1. The neck of the hernia is closed with sutures and the sac excised.
2. The stretched tissues are repaired with one of the many different materials available.

Femoral hernia

Lies *below* the inguinal canal medial to femoral vein. Commonest in females. Strangulates more easily than the inguinal hernia.

Clinical features
A swelling as in inguinal hernia, but *below* the inguinal ligament.

Treatment
Surgical repair. A truss is not suitable.

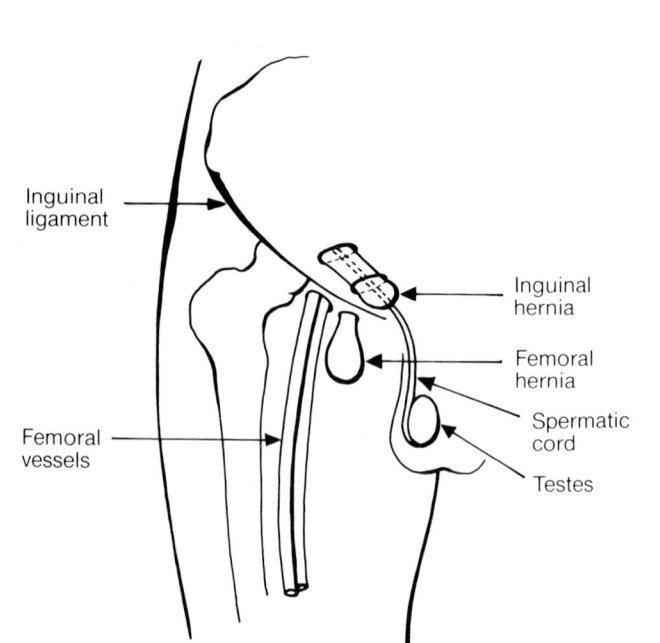

Figure 21.6
Relation of femoral hernia to inguinal hernia

Congenital umbilical hernia

A failure of the umbilical scar to fuse, and the child is born with an umbilical swelling.

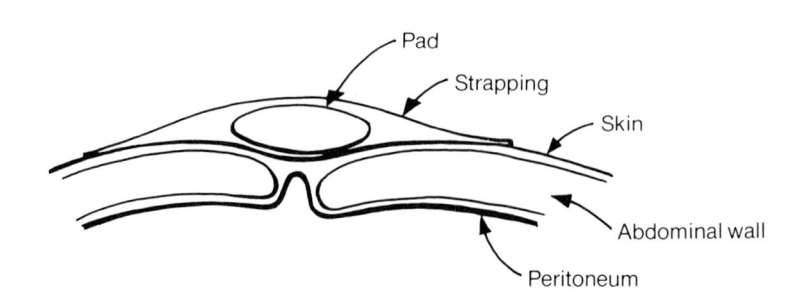

Figure 21.7
Congenital umbilical hernia – conservative treatment by pad and strapping

Treatment
1. Conservative. If the swelling is reduced and strapping applied over a small pressure pad, the majority will close spontaneously.
2. If not closed by two years, it requires surgical closure.

Para-umbilical hernia

In adults a hernia through the abdominal wall centrally just above the umbilicus.

Most are caused by obesity, coupled with abdominal muscle laxity following child birth. It can become very large and may strangulate.

Treatment
1. Surgical repair after weight reduction.
2. Surgical corset of the obstinately obese or the unfit patient.

Incisional hernia

A hernia through a previous surgical incision, usually the result of the wound having been infected.

Treatment
Surgical repair, or surgical corset.

Epigastric hernia

A tiny hernia of extra peritoneal fat through the muscle sheath in the midline below the xiphi sternum. It can be very tender as the muscles pull on it when the patient moves.

Treatment
Surgical excision of the lump of fat and repair of muscle sheath.

Diaphragmatic hernia

See hiatus hernia (p. 89).

22 Stomach and duodenum

The stomach

The stomach lies mainly in the upper left abdomen, partially protected by the left lower ribs. The cardia follows on from the oesophagus, and in turn becomes the body with an upper part the fundus. The body is continous with the pyloric antrum, which leads through the pyloric sphincter to the duodenum. Mucus is secreted by glands and by covering the surface protects the stomach from its own digestive juices.

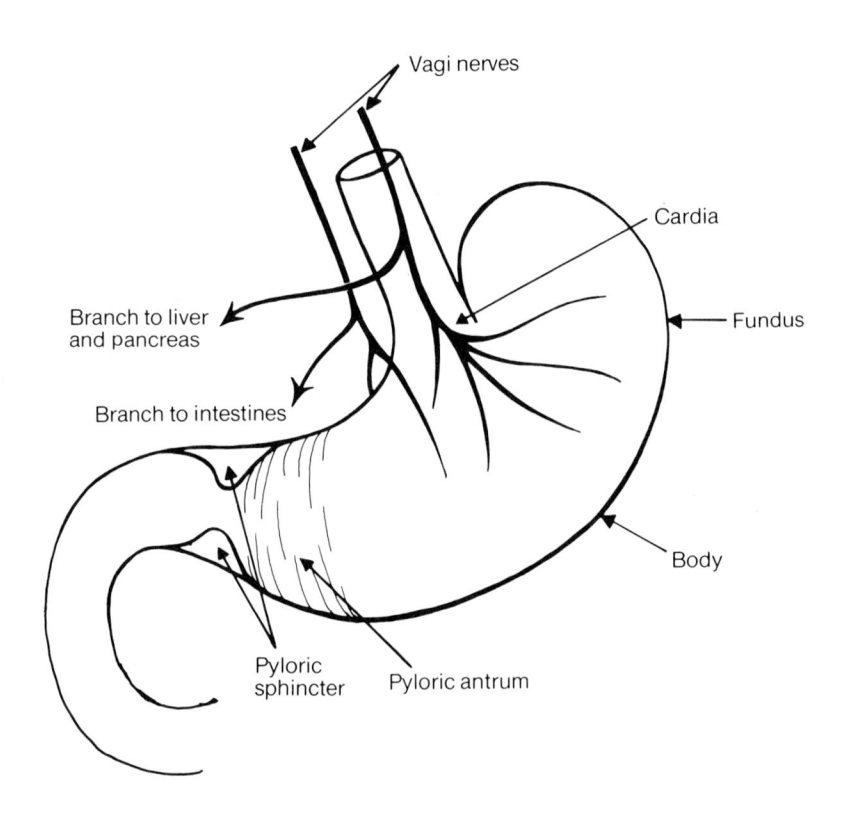

Figure 22.1 Stomach

The functions of the stomach are:
1. It is a reservoir for the food.
2. The glands secrete acid and digestive juices (containing enzymes) which start the digestion of protein and fats.
3. Muscular contractions mix these with the food, for more efficient digestion.

The secretion and the contractions are controlled in two ways:

1. Vagal. Stimulated by the sight or smell of food, the brain activates the secretions and contractions of the stomach through the vagus nerves.
2. Hormonal. Food in the antrum causes a hormone (gastrin) to enter the blood and circulate back to the stomach and maintains the secretion and contractions.

When mixed, the partially digested food is passed into the duodenum.

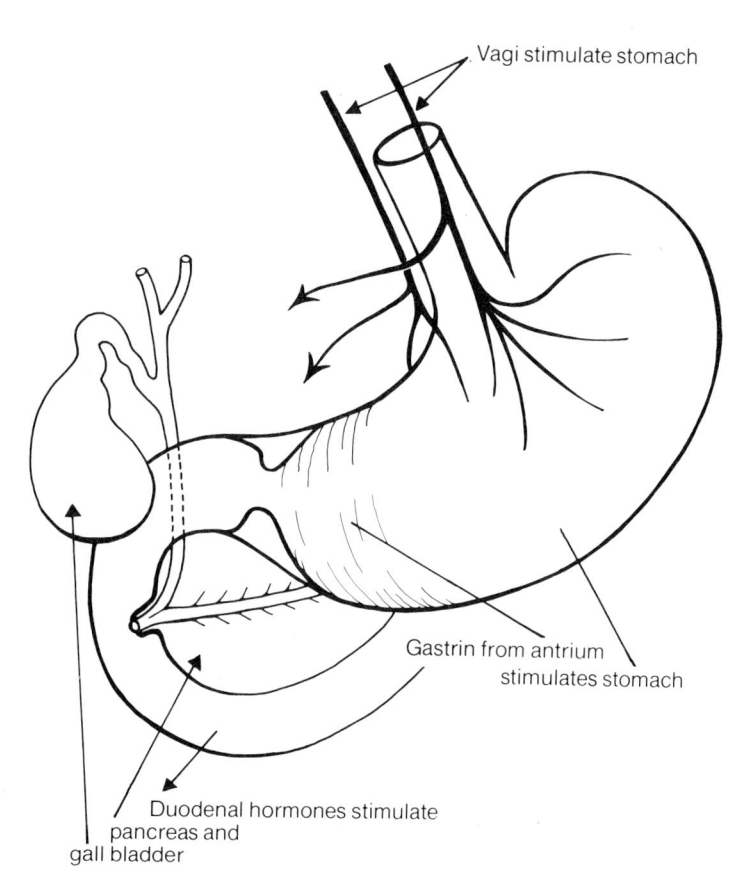

Figure 22.2
Secretory mechanisms

The duodenum

The duodenum is part of the small intestine. It is C-shaped and lies above and to the right of the umbilicus. Food in it stimulates:
1. The secretion of intestinal digestive juices (p. 111).
2. The release of hormones into the blood, which causes the production of bile and pancreatic secretions. These enter the second part of the duodenum to be mixed with the food.

Investigations of stomach and duodenum

1. *Barium meal.* Radio-opaque barium is swallowed and its course through the stomach and duodenum X-rayed.

2. *Gastroscopy.* A flexible instrument, which allows direct viewing of the stomach and also the duodenum.
3. *Biopsies* can be taken through the gastroscope.
4. *Acid secretion test* (Pentagastrin test). Stomach secretions stimulated by intravenous synthetic gastrin are collected by nasogastric tube and are measured for volume and acidity. Acid secretion can also be stimulated by causing hypoglycaemia with insulin (Insulin secretion test).

Peptic ulcer

An ulcer where gastric juice is present.
　It may be
1. Oesophageal ulcer.
2. Gastric ulcer.
3. Duodenal ulcer.
4. Stomal ulcer.
　It may be *acute* or *chronic*.

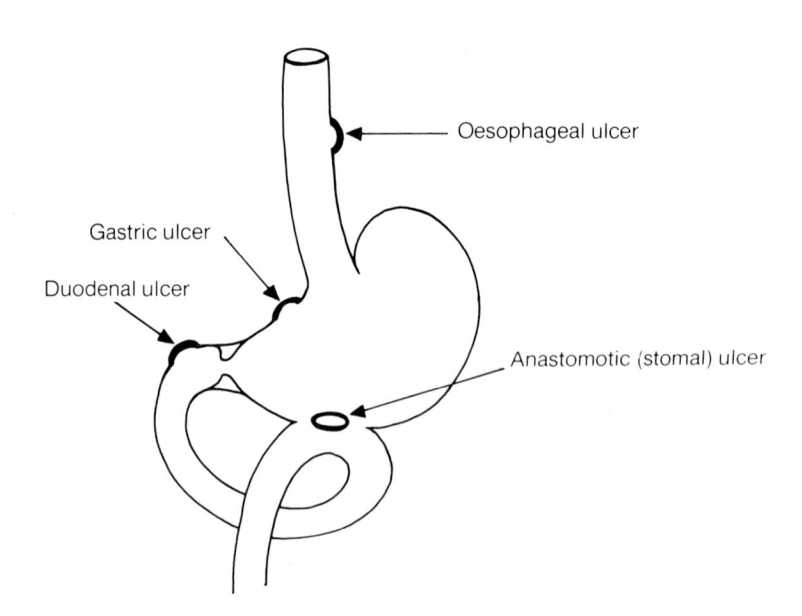

Figure 22.3
Peptic ulceration

Acute peptic ulcer

A shallow ulcer of the epithelium. Most heal quickly.

Aetiology
1. Irritation, e.g. aspirin tablets, alcohol.
2. Toxic effects, e.g burns.

Clinical features
1. An acute attack of dyspepsia.
2. Often pain over the ulcer site in upper abdomen.

Complications
1. Bleeding—haematemesis and/or melaena (p. 108).
2. Perforation—rare (p. 107).
3. May become chronic.

Treatment
1. Antacids.
2. Remove cause.
3. Treat any complications that develop.

Chronic peptic ulcer
DUODENAL ULCER
The exact cause is unknown.

Promoting factors
1. Patients of Blood Group O are more at risk.
2. There must be acid and pepsin present.
3. A possible lack of mucus protection or its faulty production has been suggested.

Clinical features
1. Epigastric pain mainly between meals.
2. The pain is relieved by antacids, milk and food.
3. The pain is relieved by vomiting (removes the acid).
4. Night pain, which wakens the patient, and is reduced by antacids.

Treatment
1. Medical
    a. Antacids to reduce acid level.
    b. Drugs to stop vagal stimulation—Pro-Banthine 15 mg t.d.s.
    c. Cimetidine, which blocks the stimulation of the acid cells by the vagus or gastrin (200 mg t.d.s).
    d. Diet which avoids irritants, e.g. alcohol.
2. Surgical. The object is to reduce the acid level.

Vagotomy
The vagus nerves are cut (truncal vagotomy), reducing the acid by 60 per cent. However, the stomach then requires help to empty as contractions (p. 103) are also affected. Therefore a gastroenterostomy or cutting of the pyloric sphincter (pyloroplasty) is added.

Recently, to avoid the complications of truncal vagotomy (p. 109), only the vagal fibres to the stomach have been divided (selective vagotomy).

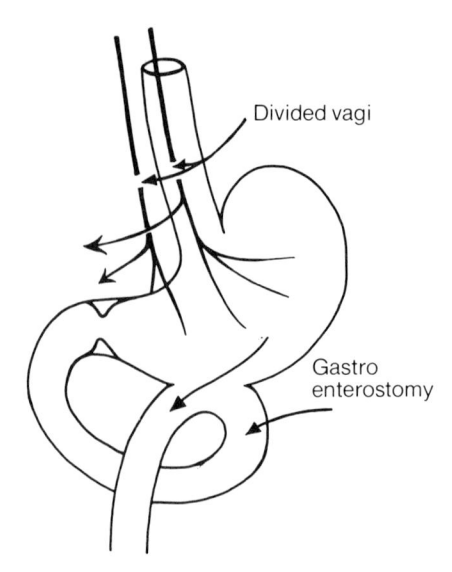

Figure 22.4
Truncal vagotomy with drainage

Antrectomy
The pyloric antrum is excised, so stopping gastrin stimulation.

Partial gastrectomy
Less commonly used now for ulcers. The greater part of the stomach is removed, so taking most of the acid secreting cells.

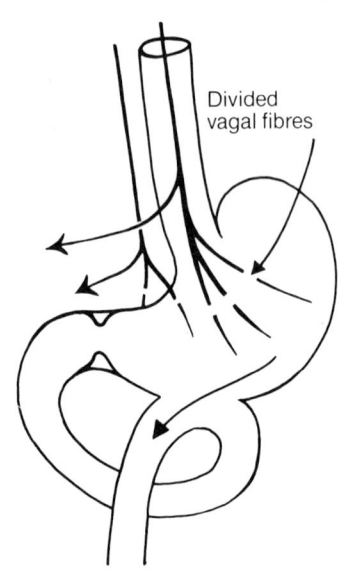

Figure 22.5
Selective vagotomy with drainage

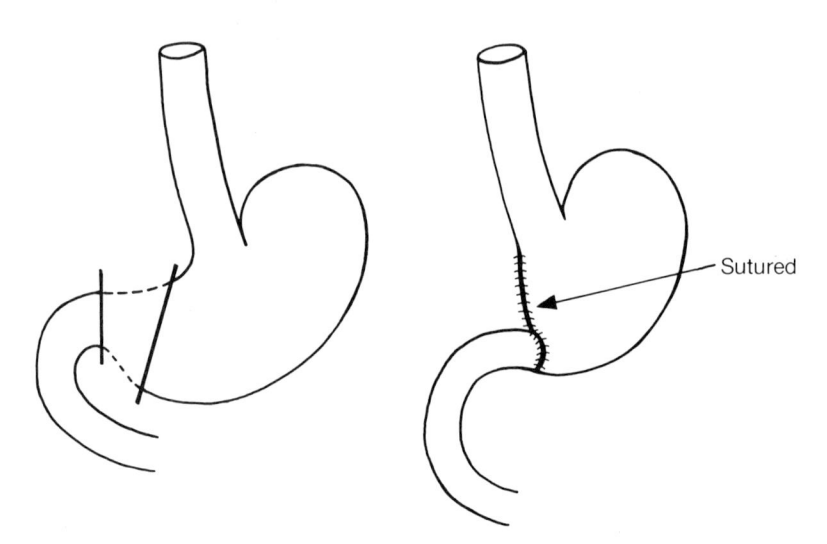

Figure 22.6
Antrectomy

GASTRIC ULCER
Found at the junction of the antrum and the body of the stomach. Cause is unknown. Associated with a normal or low acid output. Again may be a lack of mucus protection or production.

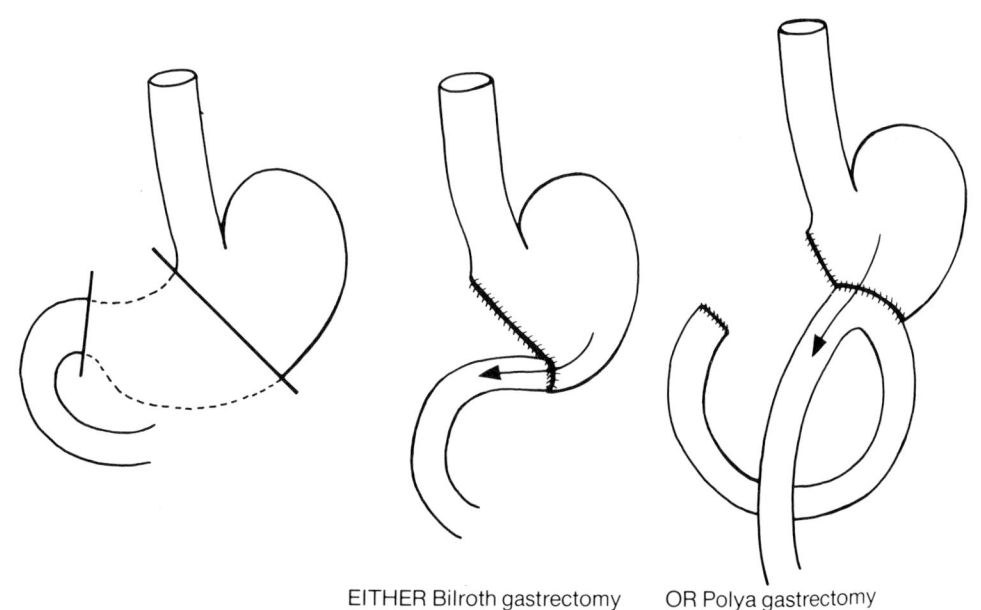

Figure 22.7
Partial gastrectomy

EITHER Bilroth gastrectomy   OR Polya gastrectomy

Clinical features
1. Epigastric pain.
2. Worse after food, (opposite to duodenal ulcer).
3. Weight loss.
4. Vomiting helps pain.

Treatment

Medical. Drugs which help the mucus protection, e.g. Biogastrone, Caved-S.

Surgical. A generous antrectomy is highly successful.

Complication of peptic ulceration

PERFORATION
Occurs mainly in duodenal ulcer. Gastric contents enter the peritoneal cavity creating severe peritonitis (p. 93).

Clinical features
1. Sudden severe abdominal pain.
2. Shock—pale, sweating.
3. Rigid abdomen.
4. Shallow breathing.
5. Confirmed by gas under diaphragm on X-ray.

Treatment
1. Naso gastric suction and intravenous drip—resuscitation.
2. Surgical closure as soon as possible.

BLEEDING
The ulcer erodes into an artery or vein.

Acute
Can be massive with vomiting of blood (haematemesis) and bloody stools (melaena).

Treatment
1. Immediate blood transfusion to combat the shock.
2. SURGERY to ligate vessels if it does not quickly stop.

Chronic
Slow ooze leading to black stools (melaena), anaemia and ill health.

Treatment
Much less urgent. There is time to correct the anaemia and then treat the ulcer medically or surgically.

STENOSIS
Chronic ulceration causes scarring, which when it contracts (p. 3) may block the stomach or the duodenum.

PYLORIC STENOSIS

Clinical features
1. Long history of duodenal ulcer, e.g. twenty years.
2. Increased vomiting, especially in the evening of the whole day's intake of food.
3. Loss of weight and ill health.
4. Electrolyte inbalance due to vomiting (p. 29).

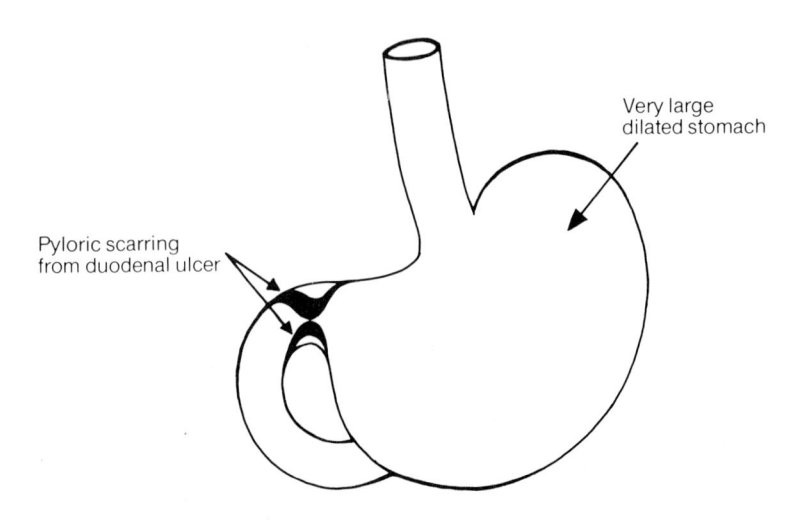

Figure 22.8
Pyloric stenosis

Treatment
Surgical treatment of the ulcer after improving the patient with intravenous fluid and electrolytes.

HOUR GLASS STOMACH
Similar but due to a gastric ulcer. The stomach becomes divided into two portions. Uncommon.

Clinical features
As for pyloric stenosis, but vomiting is more frequent.

Treatment
Requires surgical excision of the ulcer.

Complications of operation

Diarrhoea. Truncal vagotomy also divides the nerves controlling the bowel and increased motions may result.

Steatorrhoea. Bulk fatty offensive stools, which are the result of incomplete digestion and absorption of food. Truncal vagotomy is one cause, as it affects gall bladder and pancreatic secretions; see Fig. 22.1.
Both diarrhoea and steatorrhoea are avoided by selective vagotomy.

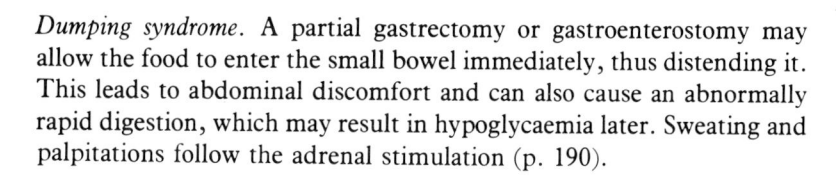

Dumping syndrome. A partial gastrectomy or gastroenterostomy may allow the food to enter the small bowel immediately, thus distending it. This leads to abdominal discomfort and can also cause an abnormally rapid digestion, which may result in hypoglycaemia later. Sweating and palpitations follow the adrenal stimulation (p. 190).

Stomal ulcer. Where an anastomosis (stoma) has been made between the stomach and the intestine (gastroenterostomy or partial gastrectomy) an ulcer may develop near the anastomosis if the acid reduction has been insufficient. Clinical features are of a duodenal ulcer and treatment is additional surgery to reduce the acid further.

Carcinoma of the stomach (adenocarcinoma)
Most develop in the pyloric antrum. Addisonian anaemia (megaloblastic) where there is complete lack of acid and often a gastritis present is a predisposing factor. The tumour spreads early to lymph nodes and the liver.

Clinical features
1. *Anorexia* developing in a middle-aged patient.
2. *Loss of weight* which may be very severe.
3. *Vomiting* may be an early symptom if the tumour blocks the antrum.
4. *Anaemia*—not only a megaloblastic anaemia as above, but an ooze from the surface can cause a hypochromic anaemia.

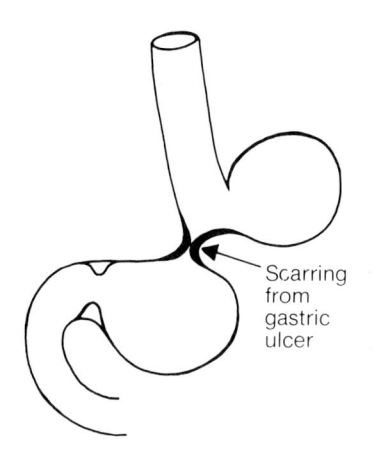

Figure 22.9
Hour-glass stomach

Treatment

Surgery
a. Low tumours: sub-total gastrectomy.
b. High tumours: Total gastrectomy.

Low tumours—sub-total gastrectomy

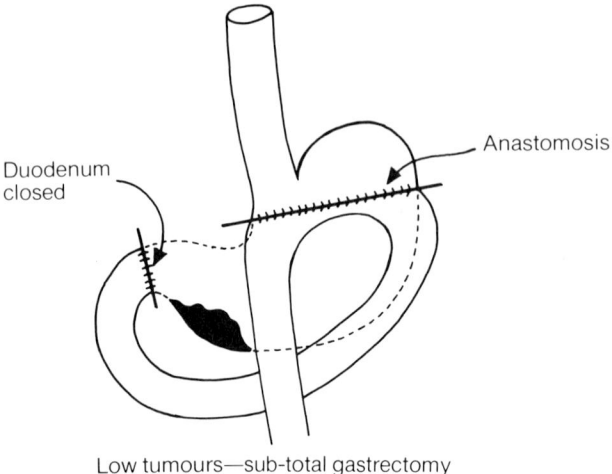

Figure 22.10
Carcinoma of the
stomach—treatment

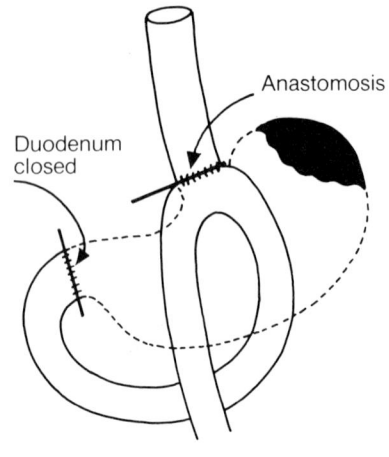

High tumours—total gastrectomy

Figure 22.11
Carcinoma of the
stomach—treatment

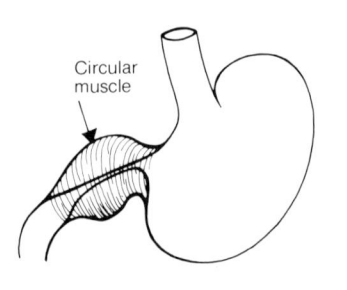

Congenital pyloric stenosis

A curious hypertrophy of the pyloric sphincter muscle which develops mostly in male babies of two to six months. Results in obstruction to the outlet of the stomach, which becomes greatly dilated.

Clinical features
1. A healthy baby starts to vomit, which gets progressively worse.
2. There is loss of weight and dehydration.
3. The hypertrophy can be felt in the abdomen as a small knob.

Treatment
1. Correct dehydration with intravenous fluid.
2. Surgical division of the pyloric muscle (Ramstedt's operation), down to the mucous membrane.

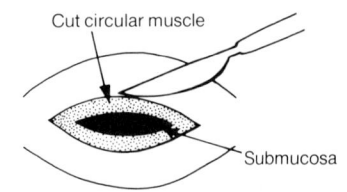

Figure 22.12
Congenital pyloric stenosis

23 Intestines

The small intestine begins at the pylorus and ends at the ileocaecal valve. It is in three main parts: duodenum (p. 103), jejunum and ileum. The intestinal secretions contain enzymes (entero kinase and amylase) which assist the digestion of the food by the pancreatic juice and bile. All the products of digestion are absorbed in the small intestine.

The colon (large intestine), stretching from the caecum to the anal canal, absorbs the fluid and stores the semi-solid waste (faeces). It secretes only mucus.

Regional enteritis (Crohn's disease)

Chronic inflammation of all coats of the gut with mucosal ulceration, usually in the last 12 to 18 inches of terminal ileum where it was first identified by Dr Crohn and called regional ileitis. It can, however, attack any part of the alimentary tract from stomach to rectum. In the colon it is often called *regional colitis*.

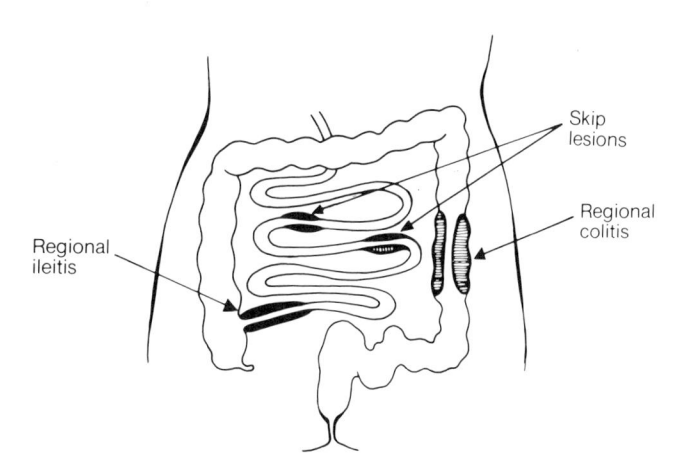

Figure 23.1
Regional enteritis

There may be multiple lesions with normal bowel between (skip lesions). Regional enteritis is a disease usually found in young people and is associated with exacerbations and remissions. The cause is unknown.

Clinical features
1. Diarrhoea and colicky abdominal pain.
2. Low grade pyrexia.
3. Loss of weight, anaemia and steatorrhoea (p. 109).

Treatment

Medical, initially
1. High protein, low residue diet.
2. Steroids help in some cases and so may a drug with a similar action salazopyrin (4–6 g/day).

Surgery. Surgical resection of the affected part, if medical treatment fails or for complications.

Complications
1. Adhesions, as a result of the inflammation as it involves all coats.
2. Obstruction, due to the lumen being narrowed by scar tissue or by adhesions.
3. Fistula (p. 4) at the site of adhesions due to continued inflammation, e.g. entero-cutaneous, entero-vaginal, entero-vesical (bladder).

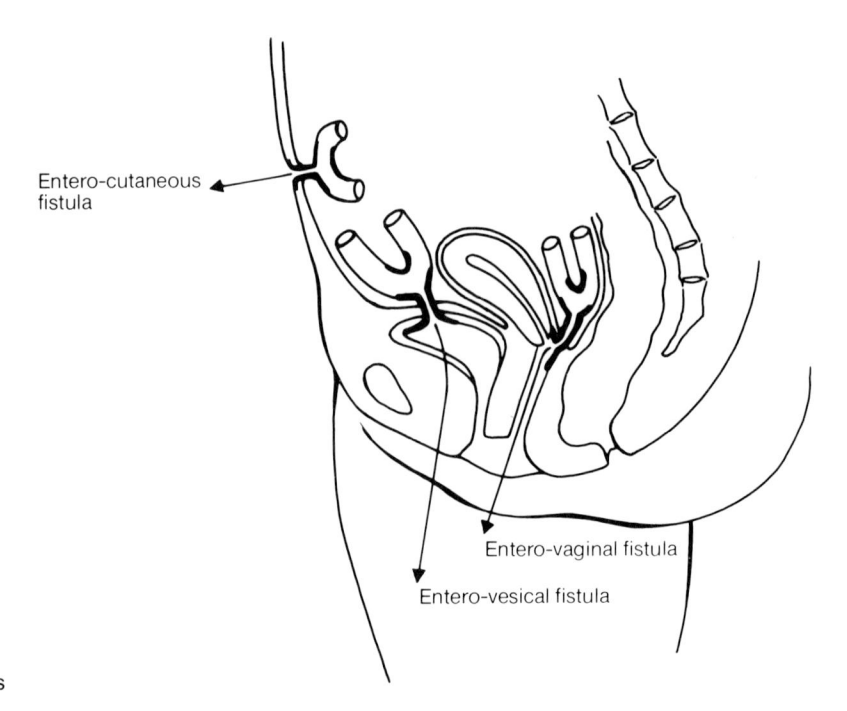

Figure 23.2
Complication of regional enteritis
1. Adhesion to other organs
2. Fistulae form at these adhesions

Appendix

Arises from the caecum and the lumen opens into the caecum. The appendix wall contains many lymph follicles. It usually lies in the right iliac fossa behind the caecum.

APPENDICITIS
Appendicitis is a disease only of advanced countries.

Pathology

1. *Non-obstructive appendicitis* (catarrhal). Inflammation of the mucous membrane and lymph follicles, but the lumen remains open allowing drainage.

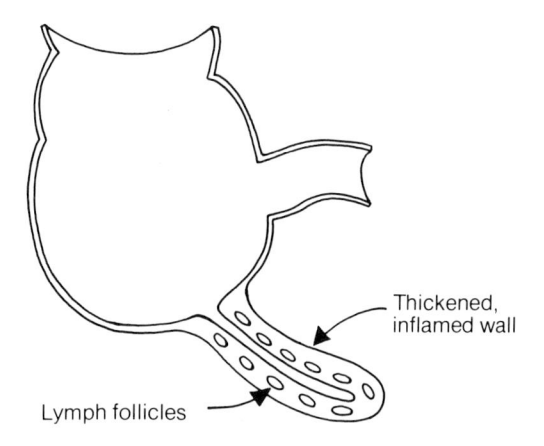

Figure 23.3
Non-obstructive appendicitis

2. *Obstructive appendicitis* (suppurative). Not only is there inflammation as in non-obstructive appendicitis, but the lumen is blocked, e.g. by thread worms, faecolith, or even by the enlarged follicles bulging into the lumen. This creates a closed cavity which distends causing gangrene and perforation of the appendix wall.

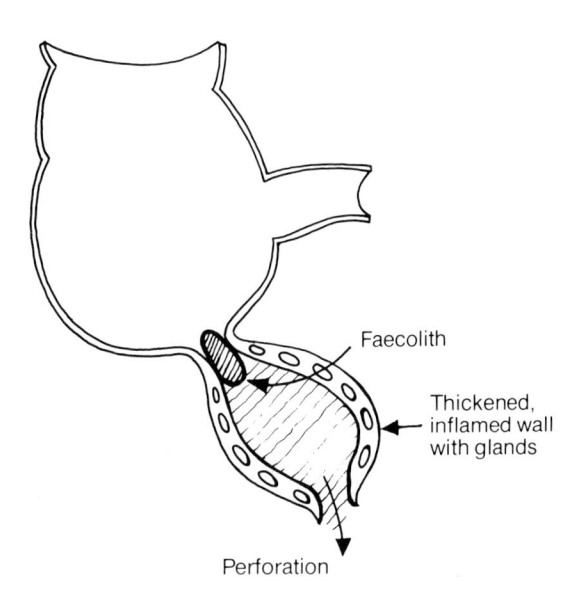

Figure 23.4
Obstructive appendicitis

Both types (but especially obstructive appendicitis) cause a local peritonitis, which may become a local abscess or general peritonitis, if not treated.

Clinical features
1. Central colicky abdominal pain from initial appendicular inflammation followed by:
2. Right iliac fossa pain from local peritonitis.
3. Nausea and vomiting.
4. Pyrexia and tachycardia.

Treatment
1. Appendicectomy and drainage if perforated.
2. Appendix abscess—drainage only—appendix is removed later.

Mesenteric adenitis

Probably a virus disease, which causes inflammation and enlargement of the mesenteric lymph glands in children.

Clinical features
It may mimic appendicitis, but the abdominal pain is usually more general. Neck glands are often enlarged.

Treatment
It settles after several days of bed rest.

Intestinal obstruction

This is the obstruction to the passage of the contents along the gut. There are two types, *mechanical* and *neurogenic*.

MECHANICAL
A physical cause blocks the gut, which peristalsis cannot overcome. It can be *acute* as with a *strangulated* hernia or *chronic* due to an encircling carcinoma.

Aetiology
1. This can be in the lumen, e.g. foreign body, gall stone.
2. It can be in the wall, e.g. encircling carcinoma.
3. It can be outside, e.g. adhesions, hernial sac strangulating.

NEUROGENIC (paralytic ileus)
The autonomic nerve supply is paralysed and peristalsis stops.

Aetiology
1. Peritonitis (p. 94). The toxins act locally on the bowel.
2. The autonomic supply can be affected in spinal injuries, uraemia and after abdominal surgery.

INTESTINES 115

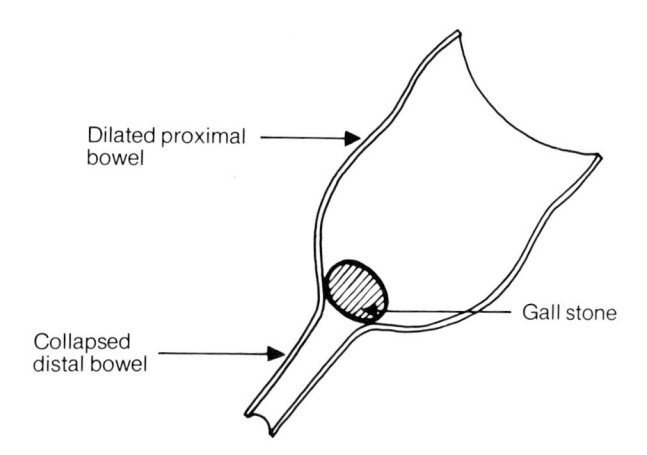

Figure 23.5
Intestinal mechanical obstruction—(1) in the lumen

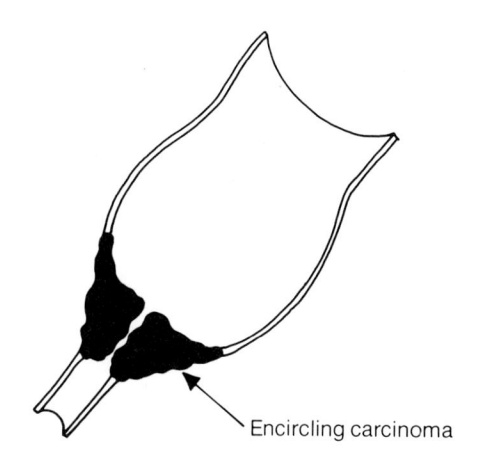

Dilated proximal bowel
Gall stone
Collapsed distal bowel

Figure 23.6
Intestinal mechanical obstruction—(2) in the wall

Encircling carcinoma

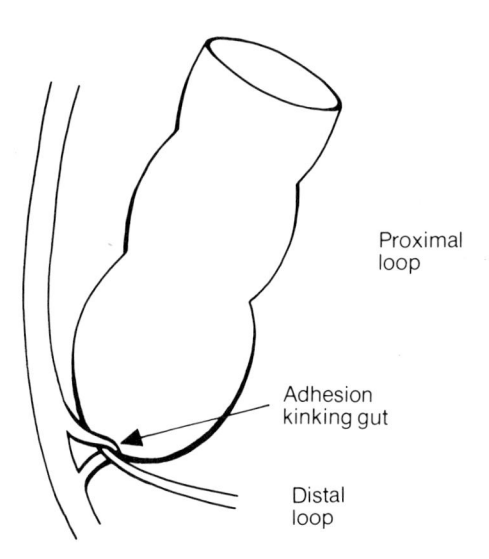

Figure 23.7
Intestinal mechanical obstruction—(3) outside the gut

Proximal loop
Adhesion kinking gut
Distal loop

Clinical features

Mechanical
1. Acute colicky abdominal pain
2. Loud bowel sounds

Paralytic
1. General discomfort
2. Silent abdomen

Both have:
3. Distension of abdomen with gas and fluid levels on X-ray.
4. Vomiting and signs of dehydration.
5. Absolute constipation of faeces and flatus.

Treatment
1. Naso gastric suction to stop vomiting and control distension.
2. Intravenous fluids to combat dehydration.
3. Surgery may be necessary to remove the cause.

SPECIAL CAUSES OF INTESTINAL OBSTRUCTION

Intussusception
A segment of bowel is pulled into the next segment by peristalsis treating it as intestinal content. Commonest in children where lymph glands at caecum push ileal wall in and it is squeezed along (ileal caecal) through the caecum into large bowel, and even as far as rectum and anus.

Clinical features
1. Usually child under two.
2. Child gets bouts of colicky abdominal pain (screams and draws up knees).
3. Normal bowel motion followed by mucus and blood from the congested mucosa (red currant jelly stool).
4. May feel mass in abdomen.
5. In the child it can pass round the colon to present at the anus as a bright red prolapse of mucous membrane.

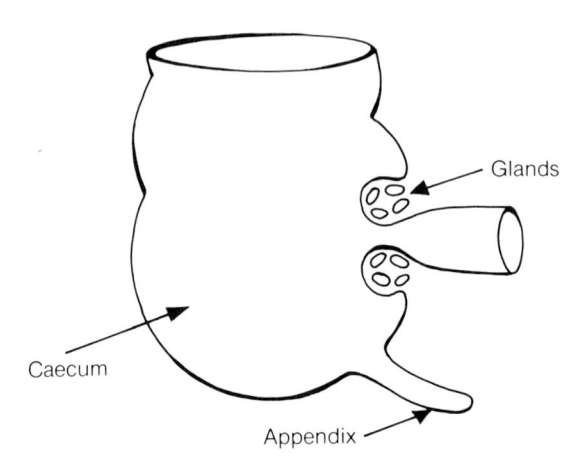

Figure 23.8
Ileo-caecal intussusception (1)

Figure 23.9
Ileo-caecal intussusception (2)

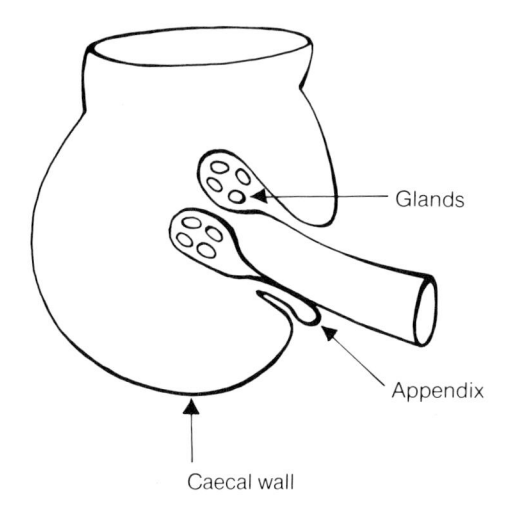

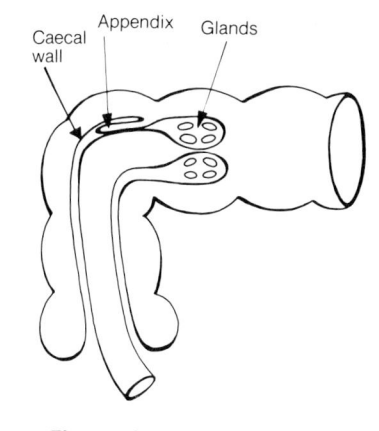

Figure 23.10
Ileo-caecal intussusception (3)

Treatment
1. Surgical reduction after 'drip and suction'.
2. The loop may have gone gangrenous and require resection.

Can happen in adults where a simple papilloma of the mucous membrane may be the cause, e.g. ileo-ileal.

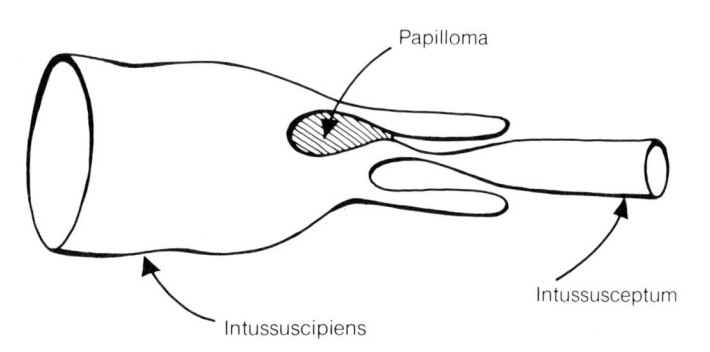

Figure 23.11
Intussusception

Volvulus
The large bowel which has a meso colon can twist on itself and so cause obstruction with a closed loop, which becomes greatly distended. It may also happen to the small bowel which twists on its mesentery.

Clinical features
Mechanical obstruction (p. 114) with gross distension of the loop on X-ray.

Treatment
Surgical excision of the large bowel loop for it may recur.

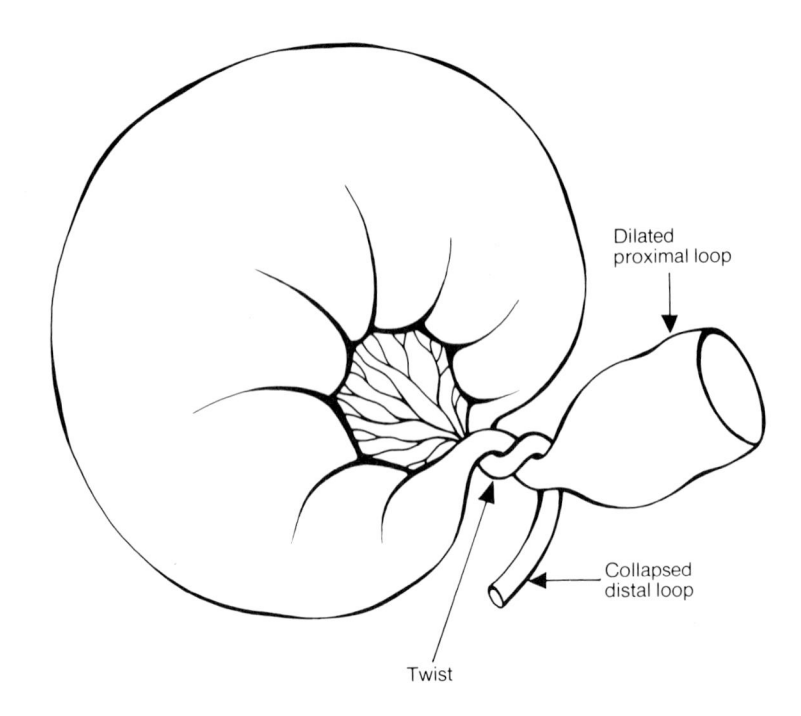

Figure 23.12
Volvulus

Mesenteric embolism (arterial)

The thrombo-embolism usually arises in the heart or the aortic wall travels in the blood to enter the superior mesenteric artery. If large it blocks the artery with resultant gangrene of all the jejunum, ileum and right colon. If smaller it travels to a smaller distal artery before impacting and causing gangrene of the supplied bowel. It carries a very heavy mortality.

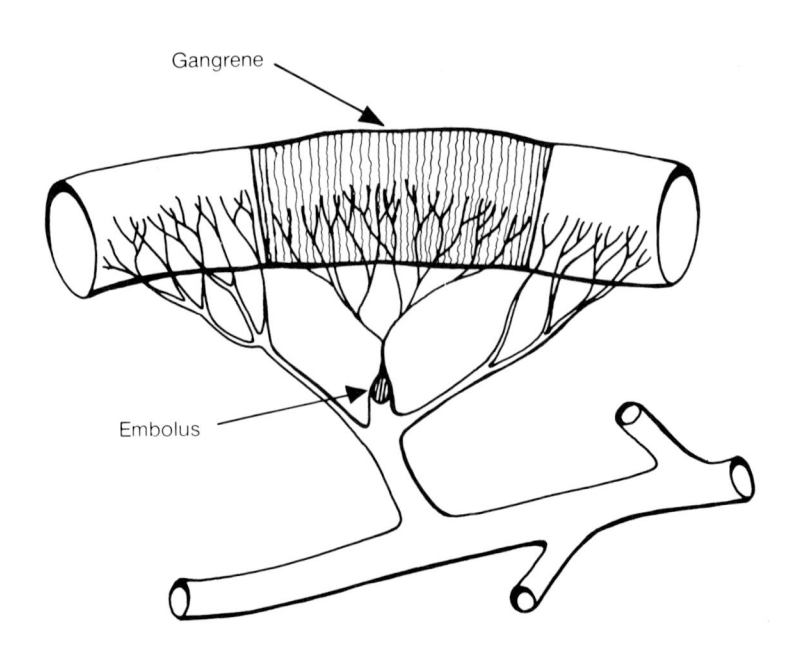

Figure 23.13
Mesenteric embolus

Clinical features
1. Severe sudden abdominal pain, often with shock.
2. Profuse vomiting, often associated initially with bloody diarrhoea as the mucous membrane dies and separates.
3. Intestinal obstruction (paralytic) only develops with the gangrene after some hours.
4. With the gangrene signs of peritonitis develop.

Treatment
If possible mesenteric embolectomy, but if gangrene resection of gangrenous bowel is necessary (patient will survive with only eighteen inches of small bowel remaining).

Mesenteric thrombosis
Similar picture to mesenteric emobolism, but with a slower onset.

Faecal impaction
May develop in the old where the bowel muscle becomes atonic and especially where bowel habit is poor as in the senile or the elderly. Hard faeces (scyballa) becomes impacted in the rectum, filling it and the colon, which becomes grossly dilated. Liquid faeces continues to enter from the ileum and flows between the faecal masses down the colon. Very little comes in contact with the mucosa and fluid is therefore not removed by absorption from it. As a result it reaches the rectum and spurious (false) diarrhoea follows.

Clinical features
1. Spurious diarrhoea with the rectum filled with hard faeces on examination.
2. May even cause intestinal obstruction.

Treatment
1. Repeated enemas.
2. If necessary manual evacuation under anaesthetic.

24 Colon and rectum

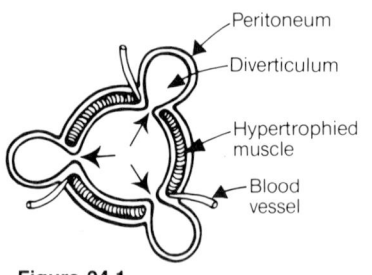

Figure 24.1 Diverticulosis

Diverticulosis

With years of chronic constipation and resultant purgation the smooth muscles of the large bowel is over-stimulated and becomes hypertrophied (thickened). The intraluminar pressure of the bowel is excessively raised by this very strong muscle. This can cause pockets of mucous membrane to blow out through weaknesses in the muscle wall where the blood vessels enter.

These are commonest in the pelvic colon. They cause no symptoms unless they become inflamed. The result is diverticulitis.

Diverticulitis

Clinical features
1. Pain and tenderness in left iliac fossa.
2. Pyrexia, often low grade and intermittent.
3. There may be a change in bowel habit.
4. Melaena—haemorrhage from the inflamed bowel.

Barium enema confirms the diagnosis.

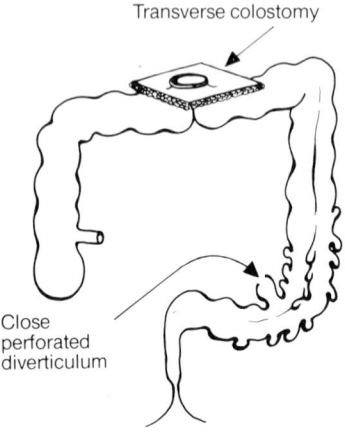

Figure 24.2 Transverse colostomy for perforated diverticulitis

Treatment

Medical
1. High roughage diet—for constipation. Stop all purgatives.
2. Bowel relaxant—Pro-Banthine 15 mg t.d.s., for muscle spasm.
3. Antibiotics for inflammation.

Surgical
If it is very severe it may require resection of the affected part of the colon.

Complications
1. *Severe haemorrhage.* Resection of the affected bowel may be required to control the bleeding.
2. *Perforation*, leading to faecal peritonitis.

    Treatment
    a. As for general peritonitis (p. 94).
    b. Closure of perforation.
    c. Transverse colostomy—to divert faeces.

3. *Fistula* between colon and another organ. The inflammation causes

adhesions to the organ and the damaged wall breaks down creating the fistula.

Vesicocolic fistula (to the bladder). The patient complains of pneumaturia (passing air in the urine). There are also recurrent attacks of cystitis (p. 192).

Vaginocolic or uterocolic fistula. Patient complains of a foul smelling discharge, often faeculant from vagina, often with irritation.

Treatment
The affected segment of the colon is resected and the hole in the other organ closed or excised in the case of the uterus (hysterectomy).

4. *Abscess.* An inflamed diverticulum may cause an abscess in the left iliac fossa.

Clinical features. As for peritoneal abscess (p. 95).
Treatment
a. Drainage of the abscess.
b. Proximal colostomy to divert faeces from the site.
c. Colostomy closed after the inflammation has been treated.

Megacolon
Grossly dilated large bowel.

CONGENITAL OR HIRSCHSPRUNG'S DISEASE
The child is born with no parasympathetic ganglia (aganglionic) in a segment of the rectum or pelvic colon. The affected bowel cannot relax to transmit peristalsis and faeces pass through only with great difficulty.

The proximal bowel becomes grossly dilated with mucosal ulceration. Many are diagnosed soon after birth by the abdominal distention and constipation, but some less affected cases remain undiagnosed till childhood.

Treatment
The affected segment is excised, but the anus and anal sphincter are preserved.

ACQUIRED
Child ignores or refuses call to stool, often due to anal pain from a fissure (p. 129). The colon and rectum fill out and dilate with faeces.

Treatment
Repeated enemata and toilet training.

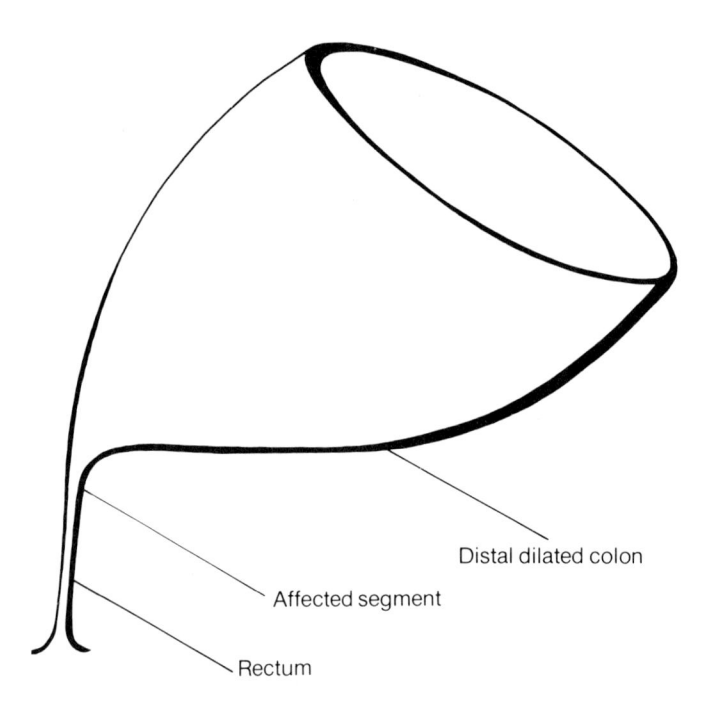

Figure 24.3
Megacolon—Hirschsprung's disease

Ulcerative colitis

Inflammation of the colon, especially the mucous membrane, usually starting in the rectum and spreading to involve all the colon, but never the small bowel. The aetiology is unknown. It varies from inflammation to widespread ulceration of the mucous membrane.

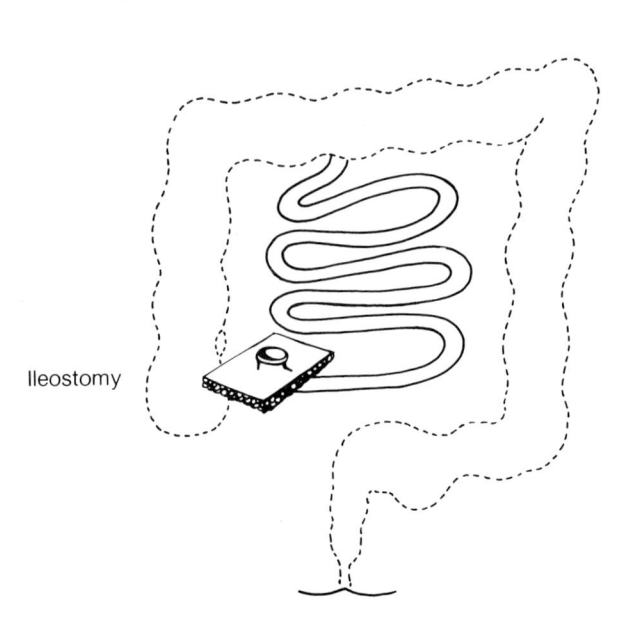

Figure 24.4
Ulcerative colitis—excision of colon, rectum and anus and formation of ileostomy

Clinical features (may be mild or very severe)
1. Diarrhoea with mucus and blood.
2. Some abdominal tenderness.
3. Chronic ill health, loss of weight and anaemia.

Complications
1. *Acute flare up.* Continuous diarrhoea with blood and pus. Patient is very ill with marked pyrexia.
2. *Perforation*—faecal peritonitis—usually the result of an acute flare up. There is a high mortality.
3. *Malignant change* may occur after some years.

Treatment

Medical
1. Steroids usually by enema initially.
2. Salazopyrine (similar action to steroids) may help 4 g/daily.
3. High protein diet and correction of anaemia.

Surgery
Surgery is indicated for
1. Failure of medical treatment.
2. Development of a complication.
3. Fear of malignancy.

The surgery is formidable, requiring the excision of the anus, rectum, colon and caecum (procto-colectomy). The ileum is brought to the surface as an ileostomy.

Tumours

ADENOMA
A benign tumour arising from the glandular epithelium of the colon or rectum, and consisting of a thin centre stalk covered by adenomatous tissue. Sometimes wrongly called polyps. They may present with bleeding or be found by chance.

Treatment
Treatment is excision, for they may turn malignant.

CARCINOMA OF COLON
Adenocarcinoma.
   The tumour may encircle the colon and cause obstruction. It spreads to mesenteric lymph nodes and to the liver.

Clinical features
There is *always a change in bowel habit*. Carcinoma of *right* colon has *increased* motions.
but
Carcinoma of *left* colon has *constipation*.

Both may have:
1. Blood and mucus in stool.
2. Loss of weight and anaemia.
3. Palpation may reveal a tender mass.
4. It may present as an intestinal obstruction.

Treatment

1. Curative. Resection of colon and rejoining of bowel (anastomosis).

Right hemicolectomy

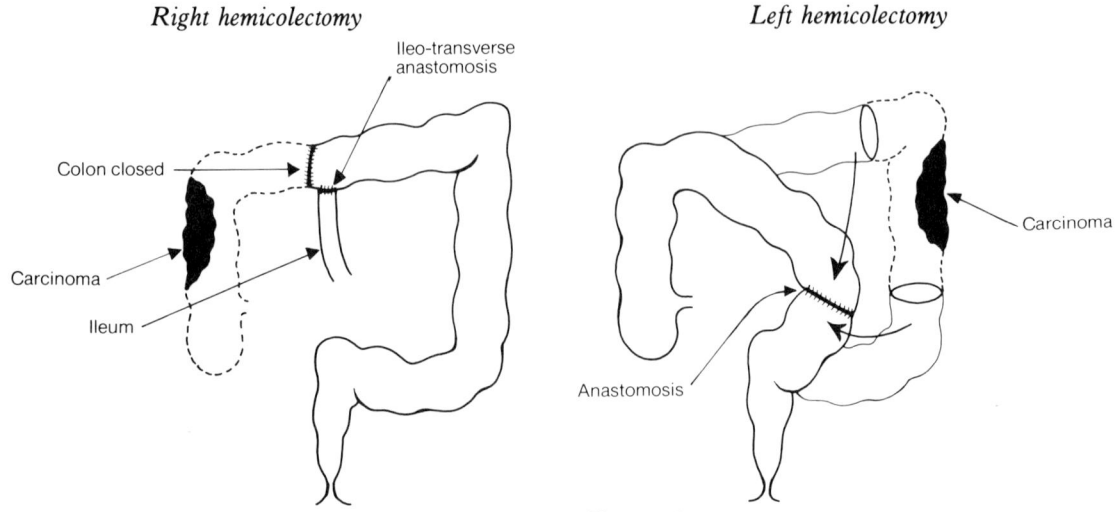

Figure 24.5
Carcinoma of the colon

Left hemicolectomy

Figure 24.6
Carcinoma of the colon

2. Palliation if tumour is inoperable. A short circuit anastomosis or a proximal colostomy will help, especially if obstruction is present.

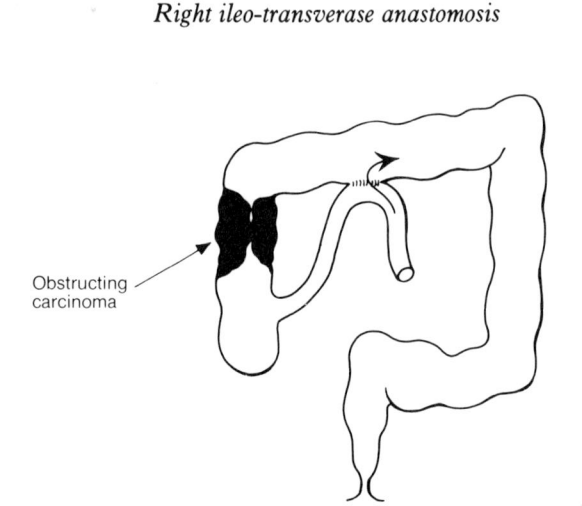

Right ileo-transverase anastomosis

Figure 24.7
Carcinoma of colon

Left transverse colon colostomy

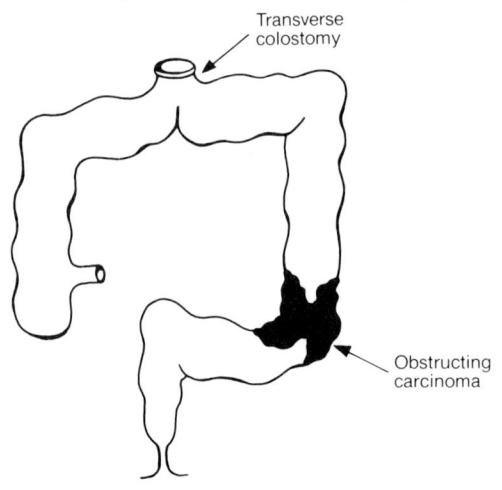

Figure 24.8
Palliative transverse colostomy

CARCINOMA OF RECTUM
Similar to colon

Clinical features
1. Change in bowel habit, usually constipation.
2. Patient complains of a feeling of incomplete defaecation.
3. Mucus and blood per rectum.

Treatment
1. If high in rectum: resection and anastomosis.
2. Most are treated by removing rectum and anus (abdomino-perineal resection) and creating a pelvic colostomy in left iliac fossa.

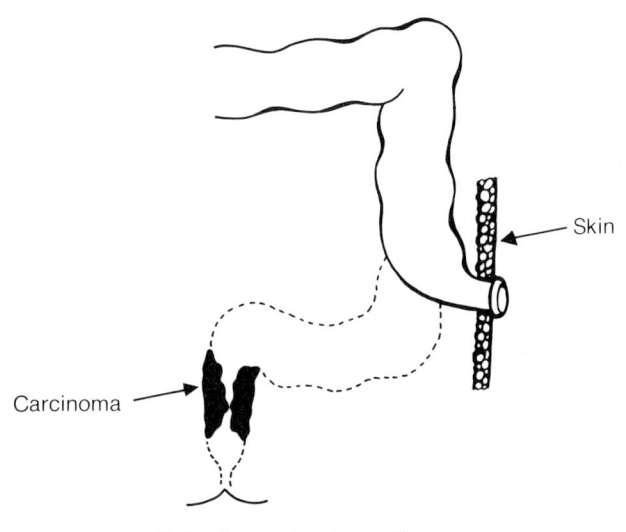

Figure 24.9 Carcinoma of rectum

Abdomino-perineal resection and pelvic colostomy

CARCINOMA OF ANUS
Squamous cell carcinoma. It spread to the inguinal lymph glands. Presents as an anal ulcer, which is very painful.

Treatment
1. Usually abdomino-perineal resection as for carcinoma of rectum, but could use radiotherapy, as it is squamous cell carcinoma (p. 46).
2. Either method is followed by radiotherapy to lymph glands.

Haemorrhoids (piles)

Dilated veins in the anal canal with redundant mucous membrane overlying them, caused usually by chronic constipation and straining.

Clinical features
1. Initially bleeding on defaecation, the straining and the hard stool cause congestion of the veins, which rupture.

2. Eventually their dilatation becomes permanent and they prolapse with the redundant mucous membrane through the anus, often causing a mucous discharge.

Treatment
1. For moderate haemorrhoids an injection of an irritant will cause them to thrombose and shrink (5 per cent phenol in almond oil).
2. Other methods to destroy the haemorrhoid are ligation with elastic bands or freezing (cryosurgery).
3. If large, then surgical ligation of the veins and the excision of excess mucous membrane.

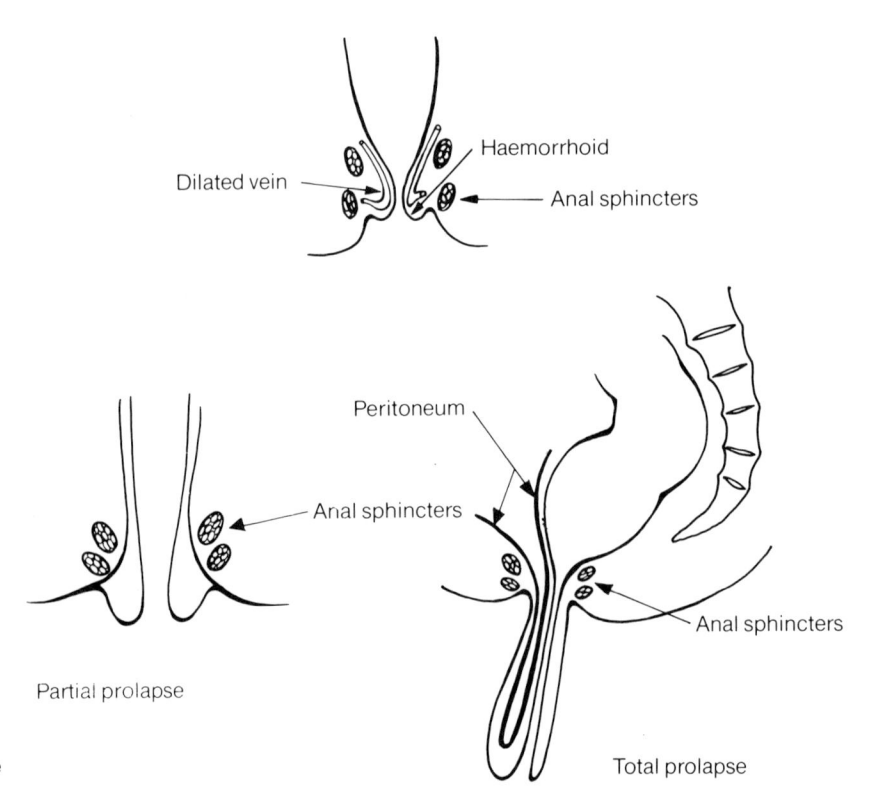

Figure 24.10
Haemorrhoids and rectal prolapse

ACUTE THROMBOSED HAEMORRHOIDS
Occasionally if the haemorrhoids prolapse, spasm of the anal sphincter prevents them returning. The tight sphincter causes them to thrombose.

Clinical features
Acutely painful haemorrhoids prolapsed from the anus.

Treatment
1. Bed rest with the foot of the bed raised to reduce congestion as much as possible.

2. Analgesics.
3. Cold packs may ease the pain until the thrombosis resolves in a few days.

Rectal prolapse

Occurs in the old where the perineal muscles have become slack. This allows the mucous membrane (partial) or even the whole bowel (complete) to fall through the sphincter. Occasionally also in constipated children.

Clinical features
Presents at the anus as a red cuff (partial) or even the whole bowel turns inside out and projects externally for six inches (complete).

Treatment

PARTIAL PROLAPSE (mucous membrane only)
Surgical removal of excess mucous membrane as for haemorrhoids.

COMPLETE PROLAPSE
The bowel is returned and a surgical repair to retain it carried out. In children it is sufficient to simply put it back, and the inflammation usually causes it to stick in place.

Bowel preparation of colonic surgery

Object: To clear the bowel of faeces and bacteria and so avoid contamination and infection of the wound.
1. Low roughage diet, reduces the bulk of the faeces, e.g. Vivonex.
2. Bowel wash-outs for two days before operation.
3. Antibiotics by mouth reduce the bacteria, e.g. metroniazide (Flagyl 800 mg daily/4 days plus neomycin 1 g daily/4 days.)

Perineal abscesses

PERIANAL
At anal margin.

ISCHIO-RECTAL
Much deeper at the side of the rectum, probably the result of an infection from anal glands.

Treatment
Surgical drainage by incision of skin over the abscess.

FISTULA IN ANO

A track from the skin to the anus. Usually the result of a previous abscess being opened or discharging through the skin.

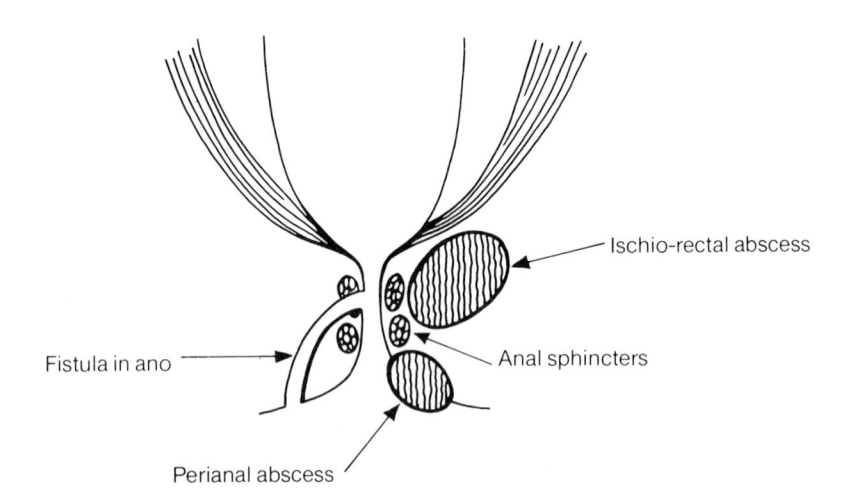

Figure 24.11
Perineal abscesses and fistula

Clinical features
Presents as a small opening at the side of anus, which discharges mucus. It often becomes inflamed and may cause further abscesses.

Treatment
Surgical excision of the tract.

Colostomy

An opening of the colon to the skin. It may be:
1. Temporary (to defunction bowel p. 121).
2. Permanent (abdomino perineal resection).

It can be a loop colostomy, or a true defunctioning colostomy. Where there is no chance of contaminating the wound, the colostomy is opened immediately after surgery.

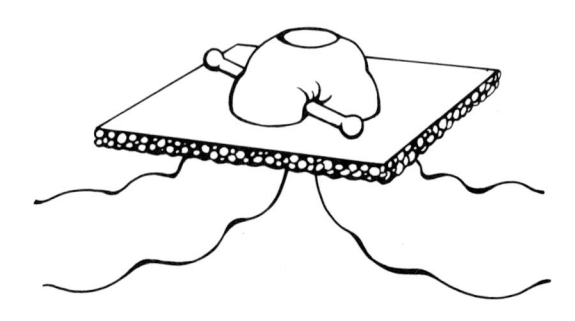

Figure 24.12
Loop colostomy

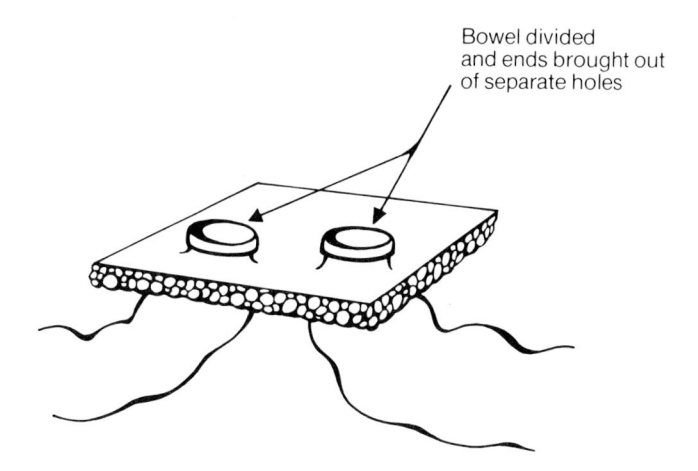

Figure 24.13
Defuncting colostomy

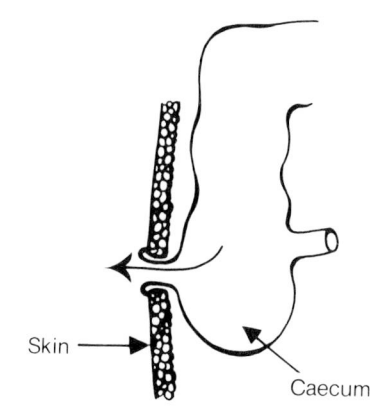

Figure 24.14
Caecostomy

Caecostomy

Opening of the caecum to the skin, which is formed occasionally in obstruction to decompress the bowel.

Anal fissure

The result of a hard stool which tears the mucous membrane of the anus on defaecation. It is intensely tender and the pain causes the anal sphincter to go into spasm, which prevents it healing.

Clinical features
1. Very painful defaecation often with slight bleeding.
2. The tender split can be seen and felt on rectal examination.

Treatment
Under general anaesthetic the anus is stretched, so overcoming the sphincter spasma and allowing the fissure to heal.

Perianal haematoma

With straining at defaecation, a small blood vessel may rupture under the skin at the anal margin resulting in a haematoma.

Clinical features
A small very tender blue nodule at the anal margin.

Treatment
1. If left alone it will be reabsorbed in ten days.
2. If it is very tender then it can be incised and the clot evacuated.

Pruritus ani

An obstinate itch situated in the perianal skin. There are many causes, e.g.
1. Irritation from sweat, dust, mucus.
2. Threadworm infestation in children.
3. Allergy to clothing.

Treatment
Find and remove the cause.

Proctitis

Inflammation of the rectum which may be part of a more general disease.

Aetiology
1. Result of bacterial infection (bacterial dysentery).
2. Result of parasitic infection (amoebic dysentery).
3. Part of ulcerative colitis (p. 122).

Treatment
Find and treat the cause.

25 Liver

The liver lies mainly below the right diaphragm, protected by the lower right ribs. The liver cells are grouped in *lobules* around a small vein, which empties into the hepatic veins. The liver is suppled by the *hepatic artery*, but it also receives the *portal vein* formed by the veins of the gut and spleen. Thus *all* the blood from the gut and spleen passes through the liver lobules before returning to the heart via the hepatic veins and inferior vena cava. This allows the products of digestion to be removed by the liver cells. These same cells secrete bile into the bile ductules (p. 138).

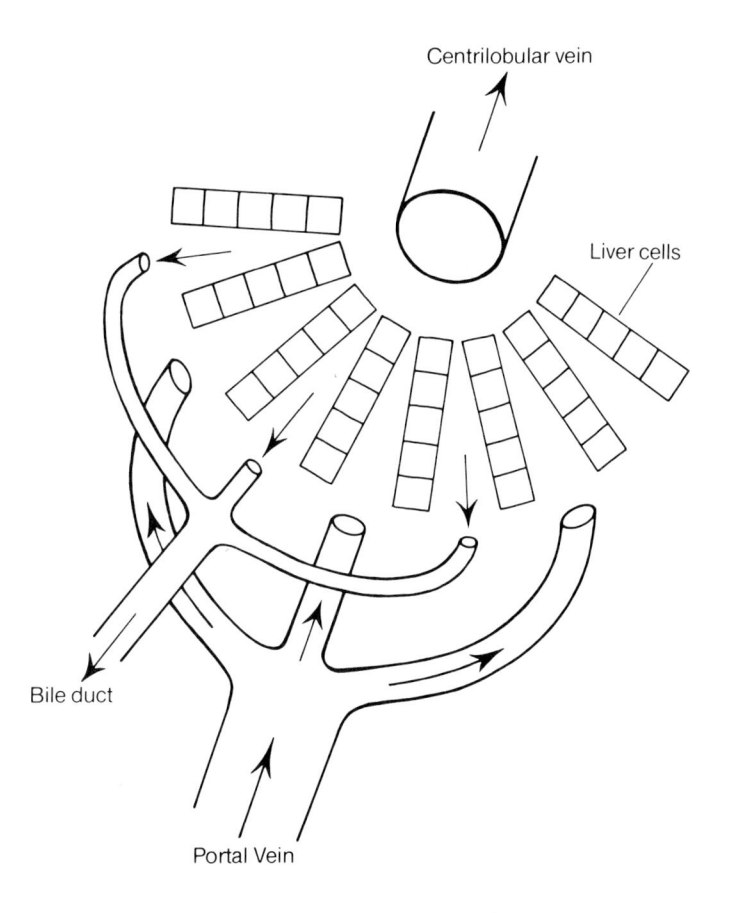

Figure 25.1
Liver lobule

Injury

RUPTURED LIVER

The result of a blow of considerable force to the upper right abdomen. The injury varies from a small tear to a major rupture of the capsule and liver tissue.

Clinical features
1. Pain in the right hypochondrium and blood irritating the diaphragm may radiate the pain to the right shoulder tip. (Diaphragm and shoulder get their nerve supply from the same cervical spinal nerves.)
2. If a serious tear then the abdomen becomes distended with blood (haemoperitoneum).
3. The patient will be shocked.

Treatment
1. Blood transfusion to combat the shock.
2. Emergency surgery to control the haemorrhage and suture the tear.

Cirrhosis of the liver

Chronic inflammation destroys the liver cells which are replaced by fibrous tissue. The liver becomes hard and nodular. The fibrous tissue partially obstructs the blood flow causing a back pressure in the portal vein (portal hypertension) with dilatation of the gut veins, especially of the distal oesophagus (oesophageal varices).

Aetiology
1. Chronic viral hepatitis.
2. Alcoholism.
3. Prolonged biliary disease.
3. Unknown (at least 50 per cent of cases).

Clinical features
1. *Liver insufficiency.* Loss of weight, anaemeia, anorexia, ascites and eventually jaundice.
2. *Oesophageal varices.* These may cause massive haematemesis.

Treatment
1. Treat any known cause, e.g. alcoholism, biliary.
2. A high carbohydrate low fat diet.
3. Surgery to prevent the oesophageal veins bleeding by reducing the portal hypertension and their dilatation by anastomosis between portal vein and inferior vena cava (porta caval shunt) which thus bypasses the liver.
4. With a sudden haemorrhage a special gastric suction tube with a balloon can be positioned, so that inflation of the balloon compresses the varices stopping the bleeding (Sengstaken tube).

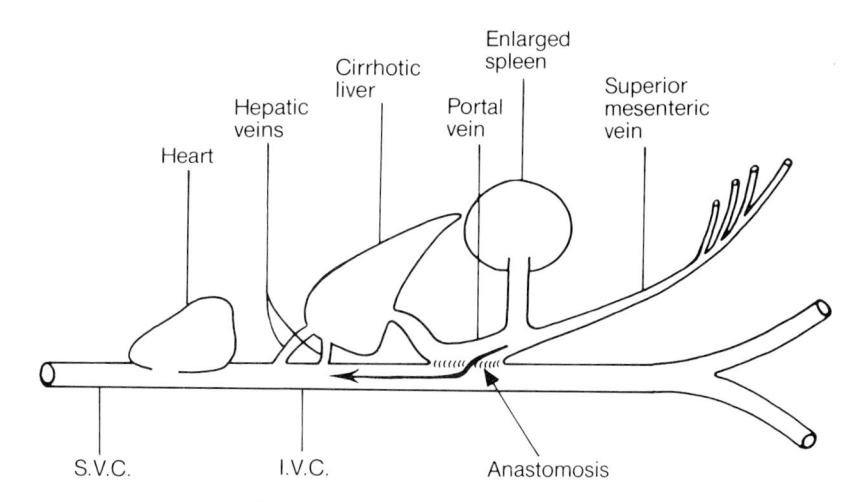

Figure 25.2
Porta-caval anastomosis

Malignant tumours

May be *primary*—hepatoma, or *secondary* metastases

HEPATOMA
A malignant tumour which arises from the liver cells. It is rare in Europe, but common in the Far East, where there is also an increased incidence in cases of cirrhosis.

Clinical features
1. Enlargement of the liver.
2. General malaise, anorexia, loss of weight.
3. May develop signs of obstructive jaundice.

Treatment
If a solitary tumour, then partial resection of the liver may be curative.

SECONDARY CARCINOMA
Liver metastases from many different tumours are very common, especially from stomach, colon, bronchus and breast.

Clinical features
Similar to hepatoma.

Treatment
Unfortunately the spread is usually too extensive. Very occasionally a single secondary can be resected.

Spleen

The spleen lies in the left upper quadrant of the abdomen, lateral to the stomach, protected by the lower left ribs.

RUPTURE OF THE SPLEEN

The result of a severe blow to the upper left abdomen. The injury can vary from a small tear in the capsule to rupture of the spleen into fragments.

Clinical features
1. Pain in the left hypochondrium and often radiating into the left shoulder tip (see liver rupture).
2. Abdominal distension with blood (haemoperitoneum).
3. Shock.

Treatment
1. Blood transfusion.
2. Emergency splenectomy.

In some anaemias (e.g. congenital haemolytic anaemia) where there is excessive destruction of red blood cells by the spleen, splenectomy gives permanent improvement.

26 Pancreas

The head of the pancreas lies in the curve of the duodenum and the body stretches across the posterior wall of the abdomen to the spleen, behind the stomach. The pancreatic duct runs the length of the gland to enter the duodenum at the Ampulla of Vater with the common bile duct. The sphincter of Oddi surrounds the pancreatic duct and common bile duct proximal to the ampulla and controls their output. The pancreas is a double gland (see Fig. 27.1).

Exocrine
Through the pancreatic duct it secretes juice containing digestive enzymes, trypsin, amylase, lipase, which digest proteins, sugar and fat respectively.

Secretion is stimulated initially the the vagus and then by food in the duodenum (p. 103).

Endocrine
From the islets of Langerhans insulin and glucagon are secreted into the blood.

Acute pancreatitis

Inflammation of the pancreas caused by the release of the digestive enzymes into the pancreatic and surrounding tissue, which they then *digest* (i.e. auto-digestion). There is wide-spread necrosis of the pancreas and retroperitoneal tissues, especially the fat, which is attacked by the lipase (fat necrosis).

Aetiology
About 50 per cent of patients have biliary disease, but the connection between it and pancreatitis is unknown. Some experts have suggested a 'blow back' or reflux of bile and pancreatic juice up the pancreatic duct and out into the tissues, caused by spasm at the Ampulla of Vater (p. 138), or even disordered peristalsis of the duodenum. Occasional cases are seen as a complication of mumps.

Clinical features
1. Acute generalised abdominal pain, which may go through to the back.
2. Nausea and vomiting.

3. Shock, which may be very severe—there is a considerable mortality.
4. Raised amylase levels in the blood.

Treatment
1. Naso-gastric suction—to lessen the stimulation of the pancreas by keeping duodenum empty (p. 103).
2. Intravenous fluids for fluid replacement and for the shock.
3. Antibiotics to stop infection of the necrotic tissue.

Complications
1. Abscess in necrotic tissue.
2. Pseudo-cyst formation—a collection of pancreatic fluid, which has escaped into peritoneal cavity and become encysted behind the stomach by adhesions.
   Treatment: It is drained at operation through an opening to the stomach which seals spontaneously when drainage is complete.
3. Diabetes from destruction of the Islets of Langerhan.

Chronic relapsing pancreatitis

It is often associated with a high intake of alcohol. There is progressive pancreatic destruction.

Clinical features
1. Recurrent abdominal pain, with often a high blood amylase.
2. Vomiting.
3. Usually a long history of alcoholism.
4. Steatorrhoea if the pancreatic damage has caused an enzyme deficiency.

Treatment
1. Stop alcohol.
2. Often the sphincter of Oddi is divided in case spasm of it is causing back pressure and reflux of juices (transduodenal sphincterotomy).

Tumours

ISLET CELL TUMOURS (from the Islets of Langerhan)
They are very uncommon and most are benign and quite small. However, because of their side effects they are serious and are a threat to the patients life. There are two types:
1. *Insulinoma.* Secretes excess insulin and causes periodical hypoglycaemia.
2. *Ulcerogenic tumour* (Zollinger-Ellison syndrome). Secretes gastrin in high quantities which stimulates high acid secretion, and causes persistent duodenal ulceration.

Treatment
Treatment of both is surgical excision.

CARCINOMA OF PANCREAS

These are adenocarcinomas and 75 per cent of them arise in the head of the gland close to the common bile duct.

Clinical features
1. Obstructive jaundice by blocking common bile duct.
2. Loss of weight.
3. There may be deep gnawing abdominal and back pain.

Treatment
1. A very major procedure of pancreatic duodenectomy, removing the duodenum and the head of pancreas, is occasionally carried out, but it has a high mortality (Whipple's operation).
2. More usually a palliative operation is used to bypass the obstruction and relieve the jaundice, e.g. cholecystjejunostomy.

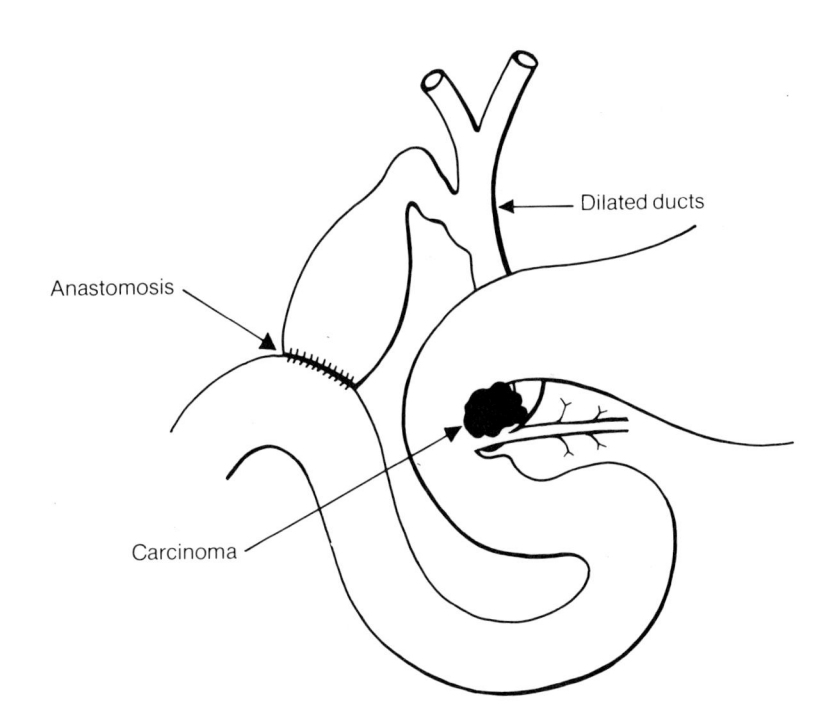

Figure 26.1
Carcinoma of pancreas—palliative cholecyst-jejunostomy

27 Biliary system

The bile ductules join together forming a right and left hepatic duct, which in turn join to form the common hepatic duct. The duct then unites with the cystic duct making the common bilt duct, which runs through the head of the pancreas. It enters the duodenum with pancreatic duct at the Ampulla of Vater, passing through the sphincter of Oddi. Between meals bile enters and is stored in the gall bladder, which is stimulated to empty by food in the duodenum (p. 103). Bile emulsifies fats breaking them into small fragments which allows them to be digested and absorbed.

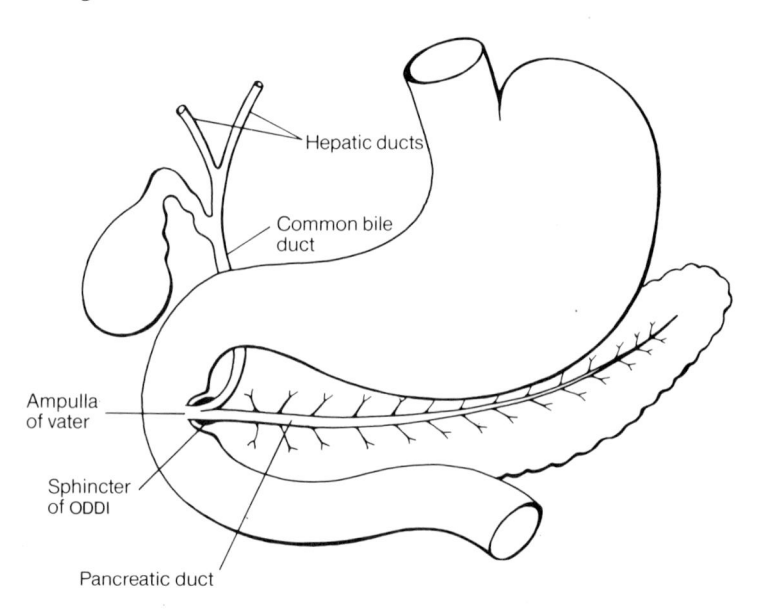

Figure 27.1
Biliary system

Investigations

CHOLECYSTOGRAM
A radio opaque chemical is swallowed, absorbed by the small intestine, carried to the liver and secreted in the bile. It is concentrated in the GALL BLADDER becoming visible on X-ray examination and so outlining the gall bladder.

INTRAVENOUS CHOLANGIOGRAM
An intravenous radio opaque chemical is concentrated in the liver and secreted in the bile. The hepatic and common bile ducts are then outlined on X-ray examination.

PERCUTANEOUS TRANSHEPATIC CHOLANGIOGRAM (PTC)
In jaundice an intravenous cholangiogram is not possible. However, if necessary a very fine needle can be passed through the skin into the liver. Under X-ray control, it is induced to enter an intrahepatic biliary duct and dye is injected which spreads to outline all the ducts. Originally, this procedure could be dangerous as it could cause an intraperitoneal biliary leak and was only used immediately preceding operation. However, better techniques have now eliminated this danger.

ENDOSCOPIC RETROGRADE CHOLANGIOPANCREAT-OGRAPHY (ERCP)
Through the gastroscope (p. 104) passed into the duodenum, a thin tube is introduced via the Ampulla of Vater into the common bile duct and pancreatic duct. Dye is then injected through the tube and the ducts can be visualised by X-ray.

LIVER SCANS
These are similar to renal scans and areas of non-function can be visualised (p. 182).

Gall stones

Some of the chemicals in the bile precipitate out under certain conditions and form gall stones.

PIGMENT STONES
Formed of bile pigments as a result of increased destruction of red blood cells in congenital haemolytic anaemia (p. 134).

CHOLESTEROL STONES
Mainly cholesterol and probably associated with a disturbance of cholesterol metabolism.

MIXED STONES
A mixture of several chemicals. They are multiple and are the result of infection.

Cholecystitis

ACUTE CHOLECYSTITIS
Acute inflammation of the gall bladder may be the FIRST presentation of biliary disease, but commonly there is a previous history of chronic cholecystitis.

Aetiology
The narrow cystic duct becomes blocked causing obstruction to the gall bladder, which swells due to the accumulation of secretions and mucin.

The commonest causes of obstruction to the cystic duct are gall stones and oedema from infection. Although not invariably, they are often present together.

Clinical features
1. Severe pain and tenderness in right hypochondrium—biliary colic (see below).
2. Pyrexia if due to infection.
3. Nausea and vomiting.

Treatment
1. Analgesics.
2. Antibiotics if infection is present.
3. Fat free diet.
4. Probable cholecystectomy later, especially if gall stones are present.

CHRONIC CHOLECYSTITIS
There is a low grade inflammation of the gall bladder wall which becomes thickened and contracted.

Aetiology
1. Infection.
2. Changes in the composition of the bile.
3. Gall stones (which can be caused by 2).

Clinical features
1. A long history of flatulent dyspepsia.
2. Intolerance to fatty foods and eggs (gall bladder is stimulated to contract by these foods (p. 103).
3. Tenderness in right hypochondrium.

Treatment
Cholecystectomy.

Biliary colic

Acute pain caused by a calculus impacted in either (a) the cystic duct and blocking the gall bladder or (b) the Ampulla of Vater and blocking the common bile duct.

BILE DUCT CALCULI
Calculi in the common bile duct may have come from the gall bladder or have formed in the duct.

Clinical features
1. Biliary colic.
2. Obstructive jaundice.

Treatment

Surgery. Exploration of the common bile duct (choledochostomy) and removal of the stones. A T-tube is left in the common bile duct post-operatively for about ten days. Dye can be injected through it and a postoperative cholangiogram carried out to confirm the removal of the calculi.

Carcinoma of the gall bladder

In the majority of cases, carcinoma develops in association with long-standing irritation from gall stones.

Presents with a gnawing right hypochondrial pain and obstructive jaundice caused by the tumour, or involved lymph nodes pressing on the bile ducts.

Treatment. Cholecystectomy, but most are inoperable when found.

28 Brain

The three membranes (meninges) which surround and protect the brain are separated from each other and from the skull by potential spaces. Through these spaces pass blood vessels and the deepest—the subarachnoid space—is filled with cerebrospinal fluid. This fluid is formed in cavities inside the brain (the ventricles) and flows out through small holes in the base of the brain into the subarachnoid space. Projections of the arachnoid mater bulge into the venous sinuses of the dura mater, allowing the fluid to drain into the venous sinuses. The meninges not only cover the brain, but continue through the foramen magnum to cover the spinal cord.

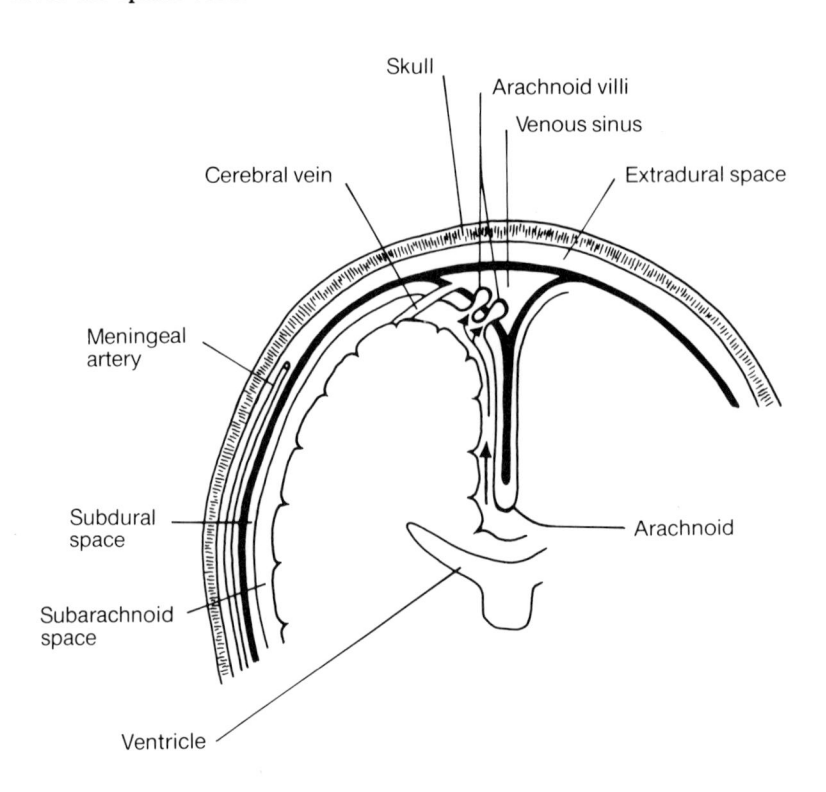

Figure 28.1
Brain

Special intracranial investigations

ARTERIOGRAPHY
Injection of dye into the carotid arteries, allows the cerebral vessels to be visualised on X-rays. They may show displacement by a tumour (p. 148) or they may show an aneurysm (p. 147) arising from them.

VENTRICULOGRAPHY
Through a burr hole in skull, air is injected into the ventricles of the brain, which can then be demonstrated by X-ray. It is used less now because of other techniques.

EMI SCAN
Multiple X-ray pictures from different directions are taken and with a computer these are turned into very detailed pictures of the brain.

ISOTOPE SCAN
Some radio-active chemicals are concentrated in brain tumours, which can then be identified using detector apparatus for radio activity (scanners).

Head injuries

SCALP LACERATIONS
After careful cleaning and removal of all debris, the edges, which are torn and bruised are excised and the wound sutured.

FRACTURES OF THE SKULL
They are sometimes associated with intracranial bleeding, but always with some degree of contusion.

Fractures may be:
1. Fractures of the vault of the skull.
2. Fractures of the base of the skull.

They can be combined, i.e. a large linear fracture of the vault may continue across the base of the skull.

Fracture of the vault

They are compound fractures where the scalp is lacerated.
1. *Linear.* There is a fissure or crack in the bone. The length may vary.
   Usually it is the result of a fall or blow by a blunt instrument.
2. *Depressed.* A portion of the skull is pushed inwards against the brain.

Fractures of the base

These are linear fractures and can also be compound by involving the cavities of the nose or ear.

Clinical signs

Anterior cranial fossa. There is a periorbital haematoma, and there may be a cerebrospinal fluid leak from the nose, if the cribiriform plate is involved (traumatic rhinorrhoea).

Middle cranial fossa. There is bleeding from the external ear through a tear in the tympanic membrane. Cerebrospinal fluid may also leak from the ear.

Posterior cranial fossa. A large suboccipital haematoma commonly forms and may present as a large, soft swelling at the nape of the neck.

Intracranial injuries

These can be divided into:
1. Injury to the brain tissue.
2. Intracranial haemorrhage.
   a. Extradural.
   b. Subdural.

They may or may not be associated with a fractured skull.

INJURY TO THE BRAIN TISSUE

Brain injury varies from mild nerve derangement and distortion (concussion) to severe tissue damage and haemorrhage (contusion and laceration).

Aetiology
1. Direct injury at the site of the blow.
2. Indirect injury. The brain is loosely supported by the dura mater and an extremely violent movement of the head by a blow (acceleration injury) or by the head hitting an object (deceleration injury) causes the brain to be suddenly displaced and distorted.

Pathology
After severe injury the brain swells from the resultant oedema and haemorrhage. This swelling limited by the skull can lead to a rise in intracranial pressure. If the brain expansion continues, the increasing pressure progressively affects the cerebral cortex, the cranial nerves, especially the III nerve and eventually the cardiovascular and respiratory centres. These centres become paralysed, which results in death.

At the present time, attempted treatments to limit the oedema do not improve the prognosis.

Signs of increasing intracranial pressure

Conscious level. The patients conscious level deteriorates with increasing unresponsiveness to stimuli.

Pupils. They start to dilate with paralysis of the III nerve then become sluggish and finally stop reacting to light.

Pulse and pressure. The pulse becomes slower and the systolic pressure rises. Terminally the pulse becomes rapid and feeble and the blood pressure falls.

Respiration. The breathing is slow and eventually it becomes Cheyne-Stoke respiration where the depth of respiration waxes and wanes and alternates with periods of apnoea (absent breathing). It is a sign of progressive deterioration of the respiration centre in the brain stem.

Clinical features

Concussion
A mild derangement of the nerves leads to instant but temporary unconsciousness. A full recovery follows with no discernible brain damage, but there is always loss of memory for immediate past events (retrograde amnesia).

Contusion and laceration
Unless the injury is very localised, i.e. direct injury, there is prolonged deep unconsciousness. Recovery is slow and often incomplete.

Treatment of head injuries
1. All patients with fractured skulls require admission to hospital for observation. Similarly all patients who are unconscious, or have been unconscious should be admitted.
2. Immediate intensive nursing is required for all unconscious patients. Respiration especially must be safe guarded and they frequently require catheterisation.
3. Frequent observations and monitoring are essential in order that the early signs of *increasing intracranial pressure from haemorrhage* is detected. It is important to get early measurements as guidelines to measure any change.

INTRACRANIAL HAEMORRHAGE

Extradural haemorrhage
The middle meningeal artery lying deep to the temporal bone may be torn by a fracture. The developing haematoma lying external to the dura mater takes time to develop, but starts to displace the cerebral hemisphere deep to it. This cerebral displacement presses firstly on the third cranial nerve of the same side and later on the other (pupillary signs). Continuing displacement compresses the brain and the brain stem, irritation them paralysing the vital centres (cardiovascular and repiratory).

Clinical features
1. A patient recovered from mild concussion becomes drowsy and unresponsive.
2. Irritation of the cerebral cortex may give twitching and eventual paralysis of the opposite side of the body.
3. The pupil on the same side initially constricts and then dilates to be followed by the opposite pupil.
4. Developing signs of increased intracranial pressure (p. 144).

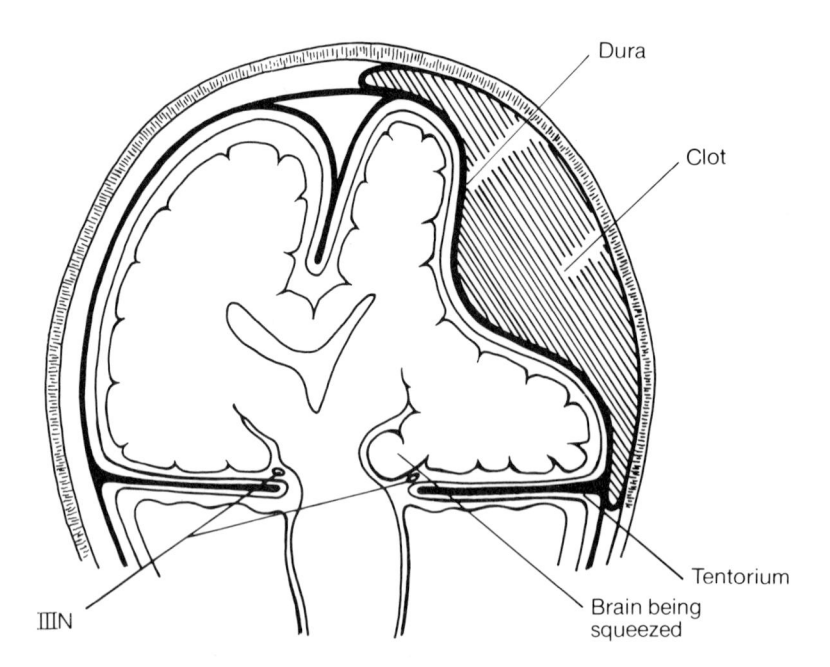

Figure 28.2
Extradural haemorrhage

Treatment
Emergency burr holes are made over the artery. The clot is evacuated and the vessel ligated.

Subdural haemorrhage
Is much more common. An injury causes the rupture of cerebral vein running from the brain surface to a venous sinus of the dura mater. The haematoma that forms lies deep to the dura mater. There are two types, acute and chronic.

Acute. This produces symptoms of raised intracranial pressure within hours or days of the injury.

Chronic. The injury may have been trivial and forgotten. The rupture allows the blood to escape and then the vein becomes sealed off. The blood clot, however, forms a cyst which expands due to fluid being drawn into it by osmotic pressure. It may take weeks to produce symptoms.

Clinical features

Acute: Symptoms of raised intracranial pressure after a head injury, and the condition mimics an extradural haemorrhage.
Chronic:
   a. Headaches.
   b. Mental slowness and apathy.
   c. Marked lethargy.
   d. Periods of unconsciousness, which get more frequent.

Treatment

Acute. Treated similarly to an extra dural haemorrhage, with evacuation of the clot and ligation of the vein.

Chronic. May require making a bone flap to empty the encysted blood.

Subarachnoid haemorrhage

Not associated with trauma, but is due often to the rupture of a tiny arterial aneurysm at the base of the brain. The blood mixes with the cerebro spinal fluid in the subarachnoid space.

Clinical features
1. Sudden excruciating headache, even unconsciousness.
2. Neck stiffness.
3. Vomiting.
4. Blood in cerebrospinal fluid on lumbar puncture.

Treatment
Ligation of the aneurysm is carried out after it is identified by investigation (p. 142).

Sequelae of cerebral injury

1. Prolonged unconsciousness
Patients may remain unconscious for a prolonged period. They will require special care, especially of respiration and chest secretions, feeding and the care of bowel, bladder and skin.

2. Cerebral irritation
As consciousness returns, the patient is often irritable with photophobia and personality changes. They may resent physical interference and lie curled up.

3. Incomplete recovery
The brain cannot repair damage. Severe head injury may be associated with permanent mental impairment and neurological loss.

4. Headaches
Are common and may persist for a long time.

5. Epilepsy
As a result of the scar tissue that forms, epilepsy may develop and require drug treatment.

Cerebral death

With intensive care apparatus, patients with *total*, irreversible brain damage can continue to function physically, for the machine takes the place of the vital centres, e.g. respiration.

Tests of the brain stem using the cranial nerves are carried out to demonstrate *no* cerebral activity. The machine can then be stopped and death confirmed.

Intracranial tumours

PRIMARY
These may arise from:
1. The cerebral tissue (the supporting cells, not the nerve cells which cannot divide).
2. From other intracranial structures.

SECONDARY
The commonest tumour is a *metastases* from outside the skull, e.g. breast, lung, etc.

MENINGIOMA
A simple fibrous tissue tumour arising from the meninges.

AUDITORY NERVE NEUROMA
A simple nerve tumour of the auditory (VIII) nerve.

CEREBRAL TUMOURS (Gliomas).
These are of widely differing malignancy.
Astrocytoma: least malignant.
Glioblastoma multiforme: most malignant.

Clinical features

The clinical features of both simple and malignant cerebral tumours can be divided into two stages.

Stage I: The tumour causes local irritation depending on its site, e.g. motor or sensory weakness, partial loss of vision, epilepsy, personality changes (frontal lobes).

Stage II: The enlarging tumour causes increased intracranial pressure displacing the brain. This causes paroxysmal headaches, vomiting, neck stiffness, drowsiness.

If this stage is not relieved, then the increased pressure will interfere with the vital centres and lead to death.

Treatment
1. The skull is opened (craniotomy) and if the tumour is simple it can be excised.
2. Malignant tumours may also be removed, or as much of them as is possible.
3. Some malignant tumours respond to radiotherapy.

Hydrocephalus

Hydrocephalus is the dilatation of the ventricles of the brain by cerebrospinal fluid, which accumulates if its circulation to the subarachnoid space is blocked.

CONGENITAL
The infant's skull has not fused, so the head enlarges to accommodate the intracranial swelling.
  There is rapid enlargement of the cranium, but not the face.

Treatment
Sometimes they can be treated by a plastic tube which can lengthen to accommodate the child's growth. One end of the tube is placed in the ventricles and from there runs under the skin of the neck and abdomen to end in the peritoneum, where it drains above the liver.

ACQUIRED
Acquired hydrocephalus occurs where disease, e.g. tumour blocks the circulation. There is no enlargement of the skull and there is atrophy of the brain. The clinical features and treatment are of the primary disease.

Cerebral abscess

Much less common now owing to antibiotics.

Aetiology
1. Previously the majority were the result of local spread from otitis media, sinusitis.
2. Most are now the result of blood spread (p. 36).

Clinical features
These are a mixture of an expanding intracranial lesion, e.g. tumour (p. 148), plus systemic signs of infection (p. 10).

Treatment
Through burr holes of the skull, needle aspirations are carried out and prolonged courses of antibiotics are given.

Pituitary gland

The pituitary gland lies on the surface of the brain close to the optic tracts. It is divided into two main parts, anterior and posterior lobes. The anterior lobe controls the adrenals, thyroid and sexual glands. The posterior lobe controls water balance, and the uterine contractions in pregnancy. The pituitary has few diseases, apart from tumours, which are uncommon.

ANTERIOR PITUITARY TUMOURS
These can have two effects:
1. Local pressure on the brain and nerves causing partial blindness and headaches.
2. *Endocrine effects.*
   a. *Hyposecretion.* Loss of sexual function and body hair, low adrenal and thyroid activity is due to the local pressure of the non secreting tumour destroying the adjacent normal secretory glands.
   b. *Hypersecretion.* Some tumours produce excess hormone which may be
      (i) Excess ACTH (adreno corticotrophic hormone) stimulates adrenal cortex and causes Cushings syndrome (p. 190).
      (ii) Excess growth hormone causes gigantism in children, but in adults where the bones have fused, achromegally (large hands, feet and thickening of facial tissues).

Treatment
1. Excision of the gland is the treatment of non-secreting tumours (i.e. local pressure only).
2. Hormone secreting tumours are usually treated by radiation.
3. Endocrine replacement with ACTH and other hormones (thyroxin) may be required after treatment.

29 The spine and spinal cord

Early in the embryo's development a groove appears along the length of its back. The groove deepens and the edges then grow across and join, starting at the middle of the back and running to both ends. The tube so formed will be the spinal cord and deeper meninges (pia and arachnoid). The tissues around it will form the dura mater, vertebrae and muscles.

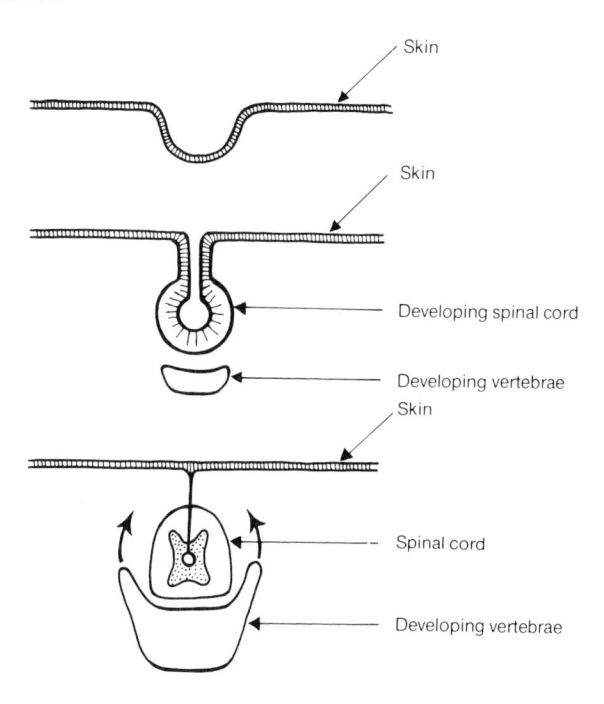

Figure 29.1
The spine and spinal cord—development

Spina bifida

In the lumbar region there may be a check to the spinal development by a failure of the vertebrae to grow posteriorly, leaving the cord and meninges covered only by skin and soft tissues (spina bifida occulta). This by itself usually has no effect, but it may be associated with failure in the development of the spinal cord and meninges, resulting in the two commonest abnormalities:
1. *Meningocele*, where the meninges herniate out through the vertebral gap.
2. *Meningomyelocele*, where the spinal cord herniates with the meninges.

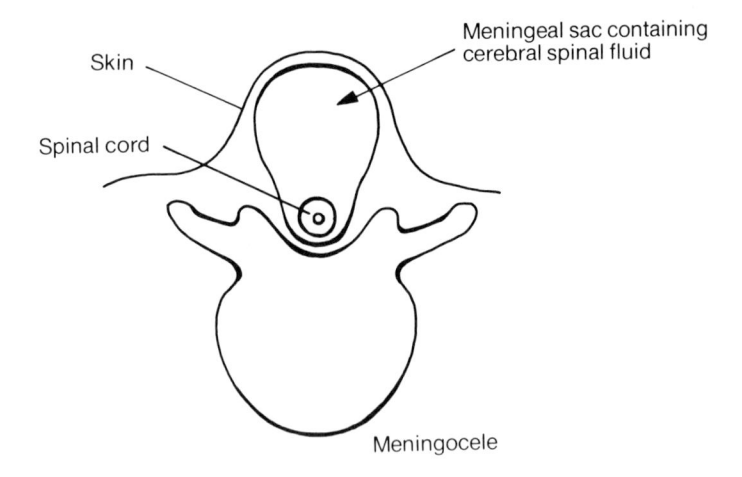

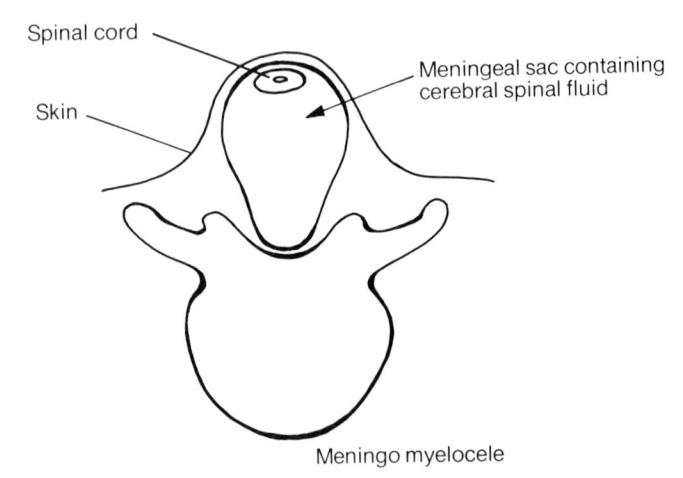

Figure 29.2
Spina bifida

(Diagram labels: Skin, Spinal cord, Meningeal sac containing cerebral spinal fluid — Meningocele; Spinal cord, Skin, Meningeal sac containing cerebral spinal fluid — Meningo myelocele)

Clinical features
The newborn child has a soft translucent swelling over lumbar spine.

Treatment
Surgery. As soon as possible the herniation is repaired.

Results
Results are often poor, especially with meningomyelocele, as these children have nerve defects causing paralysis of the lower limbs, and also of the sphincters of anus and bladder.

Injury

Injury to the spinal column may have two results:
1. Fracture of the vertebrae.
2. Possible spinal cord injury.

FRACTURES

The common fracture is a compression fracture of the vertebral body, which is caused by a severe flexing of the spine and squeezing of one vertebra between the others. A more severe injury ruptures the ligaments and dislocation occurs where the vertebrae slide forwards on the others (fracture dislocation).

Fractures and fracture dislocation may or may not be associated with injury to the spinal cord.

Treatment of spinal fractures

Cervical fractures are commonly fracture dislocations and are very unstable. The patient is immobilised in a special bed and gentle traction is applied through calipers attached to the skull. After four weeks the fracture has partially united and a plaster cast to the head and shoulder is applied.

Lumbar fractures are reduced by reversing the injury, i.e. extension of the spine pulls out the compression of the vertebrae, and the patient is immobilised in a plaster jacket.

Transverse and spinal processes

Injury may also cause fractures of the transverse or spinal processes. Although these may be very painful, they are seldom serious.

SPINAL CORD INJURIES

The cord may be injured by the fractured bones. It may be stretched, squeezed or even divided. This results in muscle paralysis and sensory loss, which is greater the higher up the cord is the injury.

The injury may be:
1. *Temporary.* If the cord has only been stretched or squeezed then the loss may only be temporary.
2. *Permanent.* If the cord is damaged then the loss is permanent for the cord cannot regenerate.

Lumbar injury causes paralysis of the legs and the perineum, including rectum and bladder.

Cervical injury will also cause paralysis of arms and even diaphragm.

Treatment

Immediate
1. Very careful handling to avoid further damage.
2. Very careful nursing, to avoid bed sores, using a turning frame, e.g. stryker.
3. Catheterisation until the bladder regains some control.
4. High lesions may require assisted respiration, although most do not survive to reach hospital.

Long-term
To rehabilitate patient with the help of physiotherapy and artificial aids.

Intervertebral disc

Between the vertebral bodies are the intervertebral discs, which act as joints and as shock absorbers. They consist of a soft centre contained within a coat of fibrous tissue.

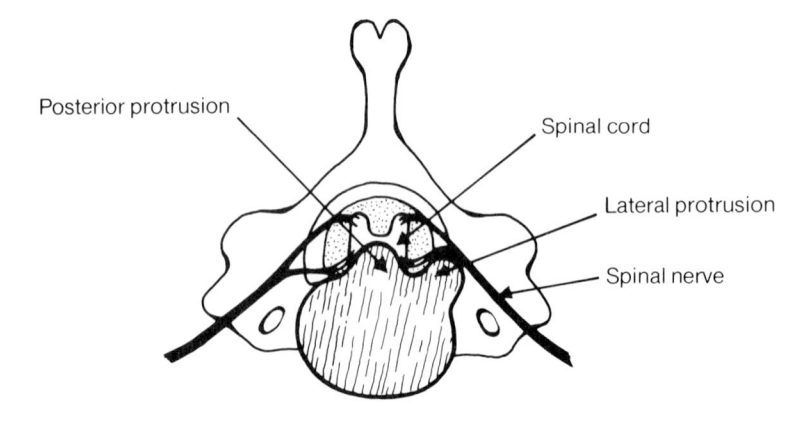

Figure 29.3
Intervertebral disc protrusion

PROTRUSION OF DISC (prolapsed disc)
Due to severe stresses and injury the centre may burst through the outer coat at its weakest points—posteriorly or laterally and so press on adjacent nerves, or spinal cord.

Clinical features
1. Pain over the spine.
2. Radiation of pain along the nerves involved, e.g. down leg (sciatic nerve) down arm (radial nerve).
3. Loss of reflexes.

Treatment
Conservative
1. Lumbar disc. Bed rest on a firm mattress for several weeks. Then mobilisation with a spinal support.
2. Cervical disc. Support with a collar until pain is relieved.

Surgery
Where pain is severe and unrelieved, the prolapsed disc is removed and the vertebrae fused together.

Other local causes of back pain:

1. *Osteoarthritis*. Degeneration of the joints (p. 172).
2. *Spondylosis*. Degeneration of the discs, which become thin.

THE SPINE AND SPINAL CORD

3. *Osteoporosis.* General thinning of the structures of the bone which may collapse as a compression fracture. Found in the elderly.
4. *Metastases.* From carcinoma of breast, prostate, lung—are common in the vertebral bodies.

Tumours of the spinal cord

Rare, but are the same types as intracranial tumours, e.g. meningioma.

Kyphosis

Kyphosis is an abnormal increase in the curve of the thoracic spine.

Aetiology

Numerous conditions (e.g. Paget's disease (p. 160), tuberculosis (p. 159) or osteoporosis) attack the vertebral bodies, which then become compressed or wedge shaped under the body's weight so increasing the natural curve.

ADOLESCENT KYPHOSIS

Inflammation develops in the thoracic discs and vertebral bodies in adolescents, and they become wedge shaped, so causing a kyphosis—round back. The cause is unknown. There is pain in the back, especially after manual work or games.

Treatment

Usually requires bed rest to remove the weight from the vertebral bodies and special plaster casts to correct the deformity. Hyperextension exercises are also of great help in milder cases.

SENILE KYPHOSIS

In the elderly, kyphosis may develop due to collapse of the upper thoracic vertebrae from osteoporosis.

Treatment is directed at the osteoporosis but a surgical support may relieve pain if it is severe.

Scoliosis

Scoliosis is a lateral curvature of the spine.

Aetiology

Congenital
There is a failure of the lateral part of the vertebral bodies to develop properly, causing the normal side to curve round the abnormality.

Treatment. There is little that can be done.

Compensatory
A short leg causes the pelvis to tilt in the erect position and the spine curves to compensate.

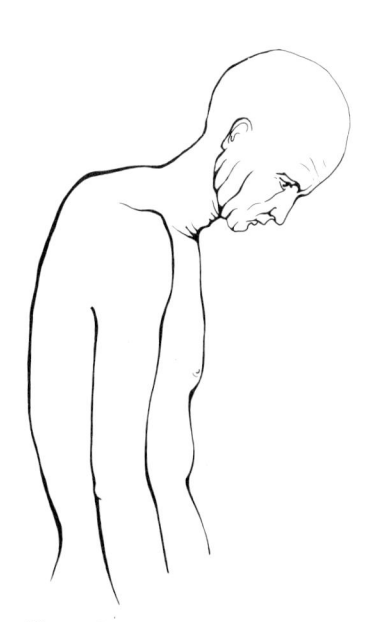

Figure 29.4
The spine—senile kyphosis

Treatment. Raising and lowering the heels of the shoes is enough in most cases.

Idiopathic
Commonly seen in adolescent girls. It may be extreme with as much as right angled deviations. Scoliosis in the thoracic vertebrae causes a marked deformity of the rib cage. The cause is unknown but is thought to be due to an imbalance of muscle tone in the spinal muscles, which maintain the normal spine.

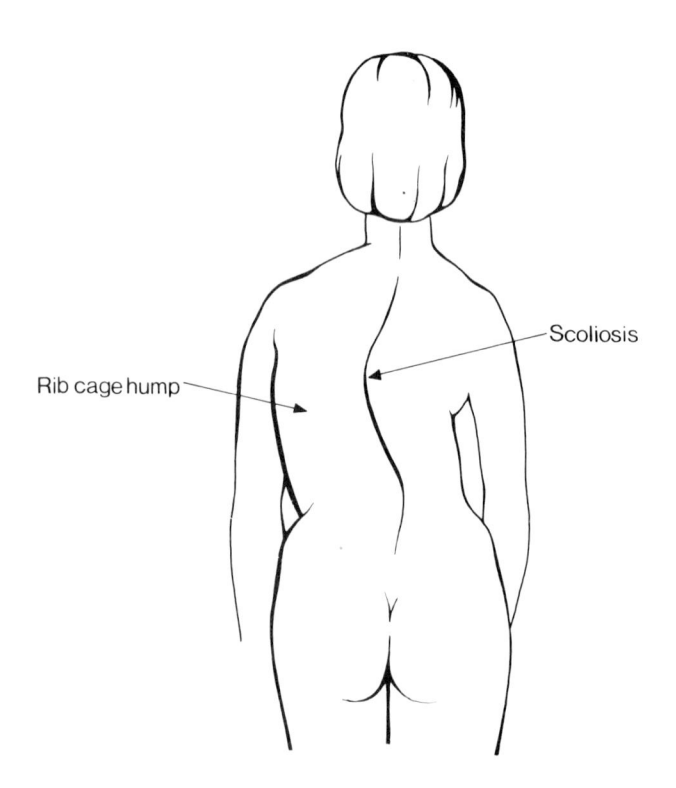

Figure 29.5
The spine—idiopathic scoliosis

Treatment. Mild cases are watched and treated with active exercises. In more severe cases the spine is gradually straightened using plaster casts. When the best position has been obtained the vertebrae are surgically fused together.

Peripheral nerves

Peripheral nerves are formed by the axons (long prolongations) from nerve cells which lie in or near to the spinal cord. Each axon is sheathed in a thin layer of cells and this makes a nerve fibre. The nerve fibres are bound together by fibrous tissue creating peripheral nerves, which will regenerate if injured. Most peripheral nerves contain both *motor and sensory fibres*.

INJURY

After division of a nerve, the distal axon degenerates, leaving empty channels, but the thin layer of cells and the fibrous tissue maintains the anatomy and the cavity remains open. Regeneration takes place by new axons growing out of the proximal cut end, into and down the distal empty channels. This only happens if the new axon can find the opening by the cut ends being close together. There is always some *motor and sensory loss*, as not all new axons find a suitable channel.

Treatment

Most divided nerves are not joined immediately (primary suture). They are left for a few weeks to allow any sepsis and oedema to settle, and during this time the fibrous sheath thickens. At operation this allows them to be more accurately stitched together (secondary suture).

Sympathetic nerve system

Part of the sympathetic system can be seen as ganglia, which are joined together and lie on either side of the bodies of the cervical thoracic and lumbar vertebrae.

These ganglia are relay stations receiving nerves from the spinal cord and sending nerves to the organs they control. The sympathetic nervous system has in general the opposite effect to the parasympathetic system.

In particular for surgical purposes it causes vasoconstriction and sweating.

SYMPATHECTOMY

Excision of the appropriate ganglia will abolish vaso constriction and sweating in the limbs.

Indication for operation

1. Extreme vaso constriction—Raynauds disease (p. 40).
2. Excessive sweating (hyperhidrosis).
3. Sympathectomy is occasionally carried out in peripheral vascular disease in an attempt to vaso dilate the collateral circulation (p. 39), and so increase the blood supply (by abolishing all vasoconstriction).

Lumbar ganglia control the legs.

Cervical ganglia control the arms.

30 Diseases of bone

Osteomyelitis

ACUTE OSTEOMYELITIS

An acute infection in bone most commonly seen in children. It is usually blood-borne from a site of infection elsewhere, and is commonly caused by *staphylococcus aureus*. The long bones of the limbs are mainly affected and the infection starts in the metaphysis (bone next to the epiphyseal cartilage plate). It may spread along the medullary cavity and through the cortex to cause a subperiosteal abscess and even arthritis in the neighbouring joint.

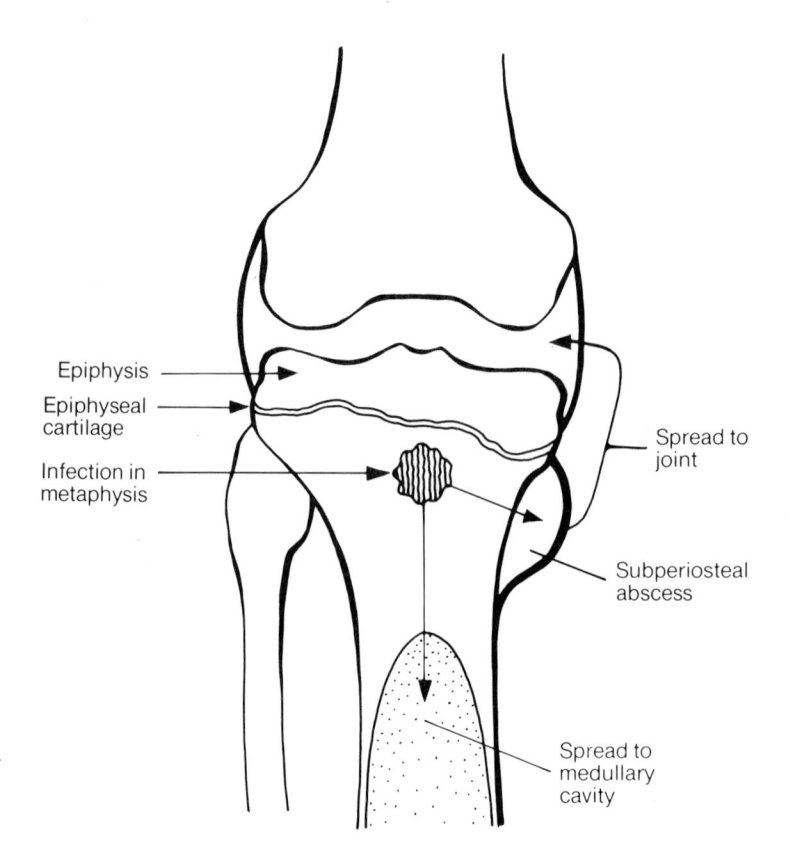

Figure 30.1
Acute osteomyelitis of upper end of tibia

Clinical features
1. Acute tenderness over the bone.
2. Swelling and redness.

3. Pain on movement.
4. Pyrexia.

Treatment
1. Prompt antibiotics, usually two in combination, will often cure it.
2. If treatment is delayed, then pus may develop, which will require to be drained by incision and, if necessary, holes drilled in the bone to allow it to escape.

Complications
1. Septic arthritis spread to nearby joints may take place if the metaphysis is inside the joint capsule, e.g. femoral and humeral heads.
2. Sequestrum formation—death of a portion of the bone. This will have to be removed surgically before healing can take place, as it acts as a foreign body.

CHRONIC OSTEOMYELITIS
Becoming rare in advanced countries.

Aetiology
1. The end result of an acute osteomyelitis inadequately treated.
2. Low grade infection by bacteria of low virulence.
3. Particular bacterial infections, e.g. tuberculosis.

Pathology
The low grade infection slowly causes absorption of bone with cavitation, abscess formation and sequestra formation.

Clinical features
1. Intermittent bone pain grumbling for a long time.
2. X-rays show cavitation.

Treatment
1. Drainage of the abscess and removal of sequestra.
2. Long term antibiotics.

Tuberculosis

Can cause a type of chronic osteomyelitis, the commonest site being the thoracic or lumbar vertebrae involving the bodies. The vast majority of patients are children. There is slow bone and disc destruction with eventual abscess formation (cold abscess, p. 14). The bone destruction leads to vertebral collapse, with resultant kyphosis and possible spinal cord damage. The abscess may point in the back or chest, tracking along a rib, or follow the spinal column, tracking in the muscle planes, to points as far away as the groin (there they may occasionally be mistaken for a hernia).

Clinical features (early)
1. Back pain and tenderness in the child.
2. Loss of movement and stiffness.
3. X-ray shows the bone destruction and often demonstrates the abscess.

Treatment
1. Antituberculous drugs (p. 14).
2. Drainage of abscess, if necessary.
3. Rest in bed until the danger of vertebral collapse is past, then probable surgical fusion of the vertebrae for strength.

Rickets

A deficiency of vitamin D in a child, causes the growing bones to be soft and easily bent. In severe cases the body weight distorts the pelvis, and the lower limbs bend outwards causing bow legs.

Treatment
Treatment consists of giving vitamin D and, if necessary, operative repair to the deformities.

Osteomalacia

Osteomalacia is similar to rickets, but occurs in adults rather than children. It is rare in advanced countries, but found especially in pregnant or parous women in countries where the diet is deficient in vitamin D and calcium (e.g. Northern China).

Osteitis deformans (Paget's disease)

A disease of the elderly. The aetiology is unknown. There is absorption of bone, which becomes soft, but simultaneously new bone is being formed, but in a haphazard fashion. It results in the bone being thicker but much weaker. The disease may affect skull, pelvis, spine and legs.

Clinical features
1. Many patients have no symptoms, especially if the condition is localised to only a few bones.
2. If involved, the legs become bowed, especially anteriorly due to the softening, and fractures are not uncommon.
3. Increase in the size of the cranium.
4. Marked kyphosis if the vertebrae are involved, leading to a great bowing of the back.
5. Pain in affected bones is common and can be severe.

Treatment
1. Calcitonin (p. 58) is now being used to halt the development of deformities and to relieve the bone pain.
2. Surgical support may be required for the deformities.

Congenital diseases

Most are uncommon and are hereditary.

ACHONDROPLASIA
Failure of the limb bones and the base of the skull, which are first formed in cartilage, to develop properly.

Clinical features
1. There is a normal trunk, but short limbs.
2. The head appears to be hydrocephalic for the skull base fails to develop.

   The circus dwarfs are often achondroplasic. A dachshund is an achondroplasic dog.

OSTEOGENESIS IMPERFECTA
The child is born with fragile bones, which fracture very easily. The fractures are a result of the thinness of the cortex of the bones, which lack strength.

Clinical features
1. The patients suffer numerous fractures with minimal trauma.
2. But very severe cases may be so weak as to die in childhood.
3. Many of the patients have blue sclera to their eyes. Gradually the bones thicken until at adulthood they are virtually normal in structure and strength.

Bone tumours

SIMPLE

Chondroma
Simple tumour composed of cartilage. Often found attached to long bones in the young where they ossify and becomes exostosis (bony projections). Occasionally they may be found in the substance of the bone.

Treatment
Local removal, if causing symptoms.

Osteoma
A simple bone tumour mainly of the skull. They are removed if pressing on other structures.

Osteoclastoma
A tumour composed of cells (osteoclasts) which dissolves the bone creating cystic spaces. The tumour is of the long bones commonly the femur or tibia and affects young adults. Most (90 per cent) are benign but some are malignant from the outset (10 per cent).

Clinical features
1. A slow growing swelling.
2. Pain may be absent or a late symptom.
3. May present as a fracture.

Treatment
1. Wide local excision because of the fear of malignancy and, if necessary, a bone graft to fill the defect.
2. Amputation may be necessary, especially if it recurs or is malignant.

PRIMARY MALIGNANCY

Osteogenic sarcoma
Most commonly seen in adolescence in the bones close to the knee, or the humerus. It is a rapidly growing tumour, which metastasises early, especially to the lungs.

Clinical features
1. Pain—may be severe enough to suggest osteomyelitis.
2. Local swelling.
3. May present as a fracture.
4. Confirmed by X-ray and biopsy.

Treatment
1. *Radical amputation* of the limb, but the results are very poor.
2. *Radiotherapy*. The tumours usually respond quickly to radiotherapy, but invariably return. It is therefore only palliative.
3. *Chemotherapy* is being increasingly used with possibly encouraging results.

SECONDARY MALIGNANCY
Secondary malignant disease is much commoner, arising from breast, lung, prostate, thyroid and other sites.

31 Fractures

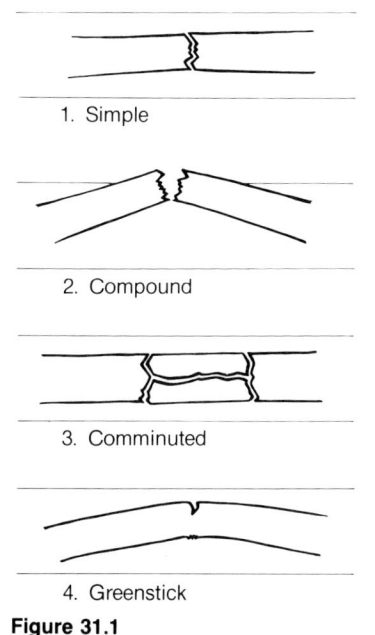

A fracture is a break in the continuity of a bone.

Types

Simple
A clean break with no complications.

Compound
Laceration to the soft tissues *exposes* the ends of the bone through the wound which may be badly contaminated by foreign material.

Comminuted
The bone is fractured into *more than two fragments*.

Greenstick
A child's bones are softer and occasionally only partially fracture and partially bend.

Depressed
Recurs in flat bones, especially the skull where direct violence pushes a portion of bone inwards.

Impacted
The fractured ends are driven into each other and become locked or impacted.

Pathological
There is underlying disease weakening the bone (e.g. metastases p. 18).

Figure 31.1 Fractures
1. Simple
2. Compound
3. Comminuted
4. Greenstick

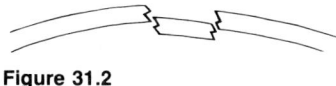

Figure 31.2 Depressed fracture

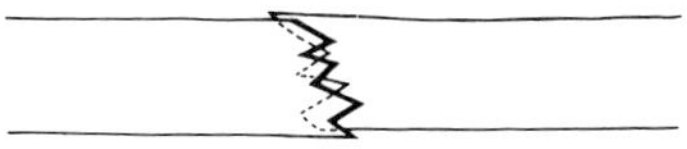

Figure 31.3 Impacted fracture

Healing
At the time of the injury, a haematoma forms round the bone ends. Capillaries and fibrous tissue grow in, absorbing the haematoma and replacing it. The fibrous tissue contains bone cells (osteoblasts), which have come from the periosteum. They deposit calcium salts in the fibrous tissue, which is now called callus. The callus is then gradually shaped to the profile of the bone by the removal of the excess by bone dissolving cells osteoclasts.

Clinical features

Not all may be present at one time.
1. Tenderness and swelling over the fracture—if compound the bone ends may be seen in the wound.
2. Deformity—there may be
   a. Angulation, due not only to the causative violence, but also to the limb muscles pulling on the bone fragments.
   b. Shortening. The tone of the limb muscles pulls the fragment and the bone ends override, e.g. thigh muscles acting on a fractured femur (p. 168).
3. Abnormal motility. The fracture acts as a false joint. Movement must be as little as possible for fear of causing further damage to soft tissues, e.g. vessels and nerves.
4. Loss of function. The limbs cannot be used.
5. Crepitus. Grating sensation as the bone ends rub together.

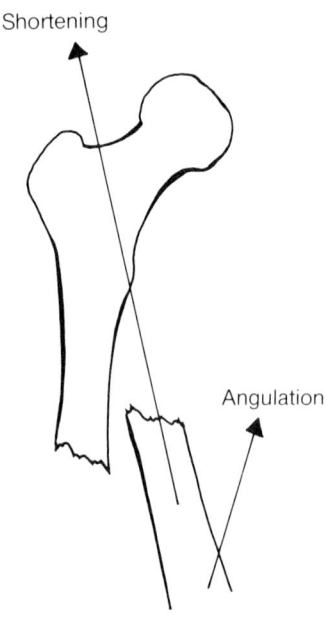

Figure 31.4 Deformity of a fracture

Complications of fractures

1. *Shock.* There is always haemorrhage at a fracture site and this may be very considerable, causing shock, e.g. in fractured pelvis or femur.

2. *Infection.* Associated most often with compound fractures, but is now uncommon.
   Prevention: 1. Prompt and very careful removal of all dead tissue and foreign material from the wound, followed by skin closure.
   2. Antibiotics and anti-tetanus toxoid.

3. *Avascular necrosis.* The fracture may interrupt the blood supply to one of the fragments which then dies. A fairly common complication of fractures of the femoral neck (p. 167).

4. *Vascular and nerve injury.* Both may be injured by the sharp bone ends. The resultant damage can lead to ischaemia of the limb and nerve loss.

5. *Malunion.* Movement of the bone ends by poor immobilisation can cause malunion. Other causes are infection and soft tissues trapped between the fragments. Eventually the ends of the bone may become adapted to each other and form a 'false joint' with slight movement (non-union).
   Malunion is treated by removing the cause, i.e. by immobilising properly.
   Non-union is treated by excising the bone ends and fixing internally. Bone grafting may be required.

6. *Pressure sore.* The result of a plaster cast or splint pressing locally with resultant necrosis of the superficial tissue (p. 165).

General treatment of fractures

Healing is helped by a good blood supply and stability of the bone ends.
1. Reduction. Any displacement or angulation at the bone ends is carefully reduced by manipulation, usually under general anaesthetic.
2. Immobilisation. To allow healing of the bone fragments together.
   a. External fixation. This is the treatment of choice in most fractures. The fracture is immobilised using external splints or plaster.
   b. Internal fixation. This is used in selected cases. The bone ends are fixed together at operation, e.g. by screws, nails or metal plates.
3. Physiotherapy and mobilisation. From the start physiotherapy is used to maintain the muscles, which waste quickly if not used. After healing is sufficiently advanced, mobilisation of the joints is commenced until the limb is fully returned to normal. Weight bearing is allowed when sufficient callus has formed.

Pressure sores

A plaster cast or splint if not carefully applied may have ridges, or local pressure areas, which press on the superficial tissues with resultant necrosis of the tissues and ulceration.

Signs
1. Persistent discomfort or pain locally after application of the cast or splint.
2. Oedema recurring after its initial subsidence.
3. Discoloration of the plaster and an unpleasant odour is highly suggestive of an ulcer.

If there is any doubt then the plaster cast or splint must be opened immediately.

Facial fractures

FACIOMAXILLARY FRACTURES
These are usually complex and may result in facial bones being pushed backwards, often as a group.

Treatment is in specialised units and consists where necessary in realignment of the displaced bones and external splinting. Most of these fractures are compound due to the nose and air sinuses being involved.

Nasal fractures
A direct blow drives the bridge of the nose into the nasal cavity or a glancing blow pushes the nose laterally. Reduction is carried out under general anaesthesia by traction with special forceps. These fractures heal very quickly.

Zygoma fracture
A fracture of the zygoma (cheek bone) is unsightly if badly depressed inwards.

Treatment
A small operation is undertaken to lever the zygoma back into proper position.

Mandible fracture
A result usually of a blow to the open and thus unsupported jaw.

Treatment
Treatment is reduction and immobilisation. This can be achieved by splints moulded to the teeth or gums if toothless. If necessary, the mandible can be splinted to the maxilla. The patient is fed by a tube passing behind the teeth. Frequent mouth washes are essential. The majority of them are compound, and infection is fairly common.

Upper limb

CLAVICLE
Commonly fractured by a fall on the point of the shoulder. It heals well and may only require an axillary pad to stop overriding and a supportive sling.

Humerus

Proximal end
These fractures heal well. After reduction a sling is enough, for it is very important to keep the shoulder joint mobile.

Shaft
These are reduced and immobilised with a U-shaped plaster. Passing from the axilla round the elbow up to the shoulder.

Distal end (supracondylar fracture)
It may involve the joint. There is a real danger of the brachial artery being damaged. After reduction the arm is immobilised at right angles in a plaster cast, and the patient admitted for observation to ensure the blood supply to the distal limb has not been jeopardised.

Radial head
A small crack is treated simply by immobilisation of the arm in a sling for two to three weeks.

A more serious fracture with fragmentation is best treated by excision of the head which can now be replaced by one of plastic.

Ulna
Olecranon process. This requires to be screwed back on.

Forearm

Fracture of one bone can be reduced using the other as a splint. Fracture of both bones is much more difficult and may require internal fixation by a metal plate.

Wrist (Colles' fracture)

Very common. The main injury is a fracture of the lower end of radius which is pushed dorsally, resulting in a 'dinner fork' deformity. Reduction is followed by a plaster cast from forearm to the middle of the palm.

Carpal

Any of these can be fractured but the commonest is the scaphoid. This requires absolute immobilisation often for a long time in plaster from forearm to mid-palm.

Metacarpals

If necessary the fracture is reduced. A plaster of paris mould (back slab) is applied to the dorsum of the hand for three to four weeks.

A fracture of the thumb (1st) metacarpal may involve the carpal—metacarpal joints (Bennett's fracture). It is treated most carefully by reduction and fixation to avoid stiffness and disability of the thumb in the future from osteoarthritis (p. 172).

Phalanges

After reduction, it can be strapped to its neighbour, which acts as a splint or a small plaster cast can be used.

Lower limb

PELVIS

Most fractures involve the pelvic rami and there is often damage to soft tissues, e.g. urethra (p. 201). There is considerable haemorrhage and the patient is often shocked.

Apart from treatment of the shock and other injuries the fracture is treated by simple support. This can be obtained simply by immobilisation in bed between sand bags.

FEMUR

Head and neck

There are two main sites for fracture.
1. The femoral neck (cervical fracture).
2. At the junction of the neck and shaft (intertrochanteric fracture).
Both are treated initially by internal fixation with a nail (Smith Petersen) and a supporting plate (intertrochanteric).

The blood supply to the femoral head in cervical fractures is frequently insufficient and it can develop avascular necrosis (p. 164). Should this happen it is excised and replaced by an artificial head, or even the whole joint is replaced, i.e. head of femur and acetabulum.

Increasingly prothesis (artificial heads of femur and joints) are being used as the initial treatment of fractures of the femoral neck.

Shaft and distal end

External fixation is used where internal fixation is not specially indicated. But the soft bulk of the thigh makes immobilisation in a plaster cast impractical, for the bone ends would override causing shortening. This is prevented by traction where the distal fragment is pulled gently either by strapping (skin traction) or by a pin through the distal fragment or tibial tuberosity (skeletal traction).

The counter pull can be obtained by
1. Using a Thomas Splint, the padded ring of which presses against the ischial spine (fixed traction).
2. Tilting the bed and using the patients weight (sliding traction).

The leg being supported on a splint, which also prevents angulation.

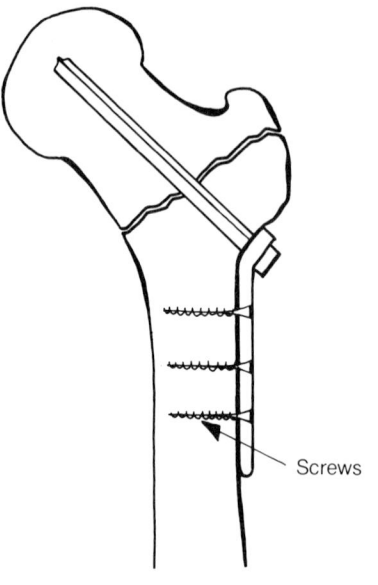

Figure 31.5
Nail and plate for intertrochanteric fracture of femur

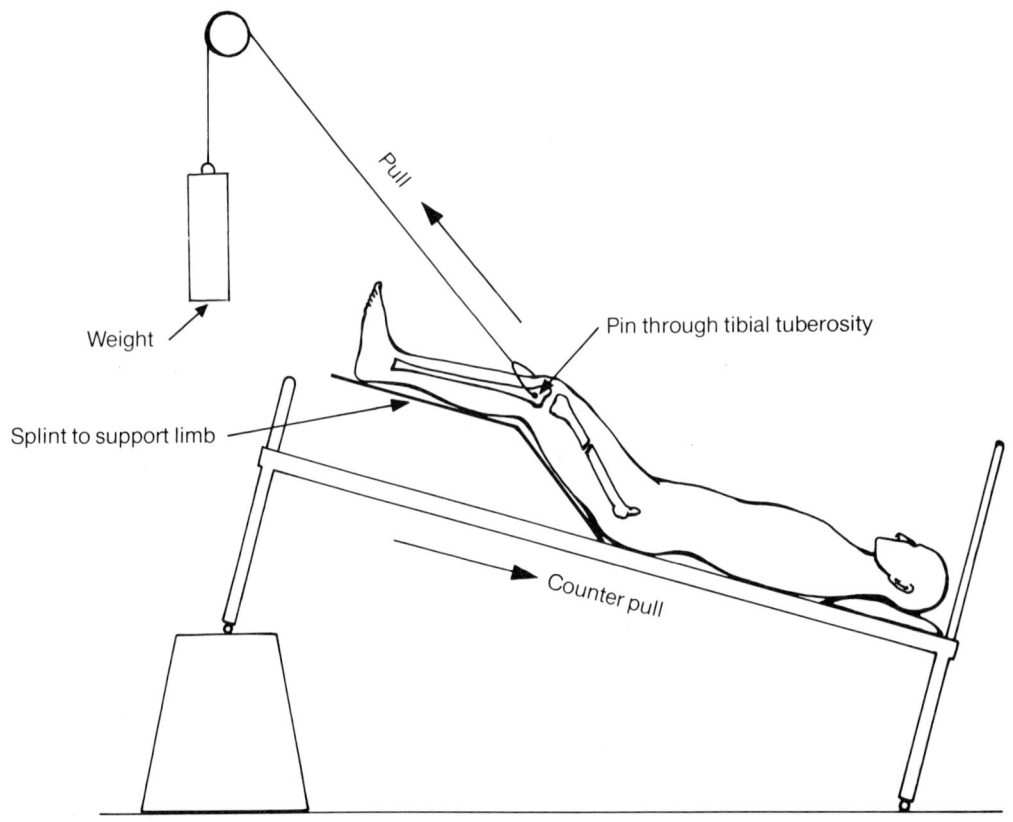

Figure 31.6
Balanced traction for fractured femoral shaft

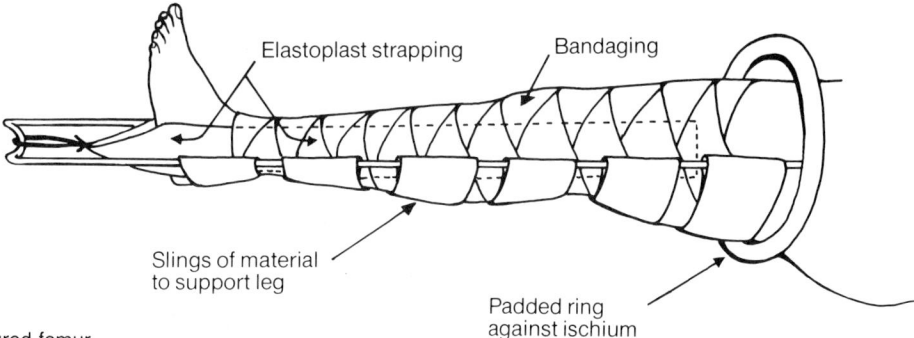

Figure 31.7
Thomas splint for fractured femur

Internal fixation is sometimes employed for simple fractures and also where angulation is severe. It can be a metal plate across the fracture site, or a large nail in the medullary cavity (Kuntschner nail).

Patella
Fractures can be treated by internal fixation, but usually the fragments are excised, for it avoids osteoarthritis developing later, but the excision gives an unsightly appearance.

TIBIA

Proximal end
The commonest fracture is displacement of the lateral condyle caused by a blow angling the knee joint and tearing the medial ligaments of the joint.

To avoid osteoarthritis in the future, accurate reduction is essential and is best obtained by internal fixation of the condyle by a screw. The joint is immobilised by a plaster cast for several weeks to allow healing of the ligaments.

In elderly patients a degree of displacement may be accepted in order to get early mobilisation.

Shaft
These are often compound and involve both bones.

If easily reduced, then it is immobilised in a plaster cast from mid-thigh to toes and if the fibula is not broken, it acts as an additional splint. With a fracture that is unstable and the possibility of overriding, internal fixation is used.

This is not possible where the fracture is compound and external fixation is required along with traction by a pin through the calcaneum.

Distal end
There are a number of different types of fracture of the tibia and fibula at the ankle joint. Fractures that involve the malleoli cause the ankle joint to become unstable and to dislocate. This condition is a fracture dislocation (Pott's fracture). These are often treated by internal fixation

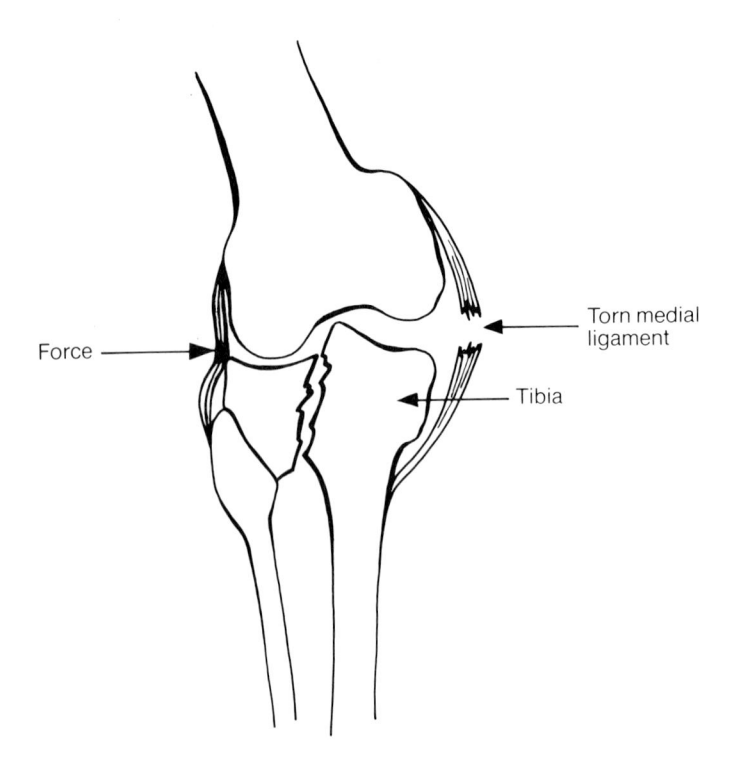

Figure 31.8
Fracture of upper end of tibia

of the malleoli to stabilise the joint and a plaster cast to allow the ligaments to heal. Some can be treated by reduction and external fixation by a plaster cast only.

Tarsal bones
Fractures are unusual and are most often caused by landing on the feet from a high fall (e.g. parachuting). The bones are crushed by the patients weight. They are treated by reduction if necessary and a plaster cast.

Metatarsals
These may be fractured by crushing, e.g. by a weight or occasionally they fracture spontaneously when walking on rough ground (march fracture). Any displacement is reduced and a plaster cast, which allows walking, protects it and is the most comfortable treatment.

Phalanges
Fractures are caused mainly by crushing and most are treated by strapping.

32 Joints

There are various types of joints, but the synovial joint is of most surgical interest. The articular surfaces are of hyaline cartilages and the joint is held in place by a capsule supported by surrounding ligaments and muscles. The capsule is lined by synovial membrane, which secretes synovial fluid, which lubricates and nourishes the articular cartilage layers.

Arthritis

ACUTE ARTHRITIS
Acute inflammation of the joints causes an outpouring of synovial fluid (effusion) from the inflamed synovia. It may be blood stained (haemarthrosis) if associated with trauma.

Aetiology
1. Infection. Acute pyogenic arthritis is usually caused by the staphylococcus or the streptococcus.
    The possible routes of infection are:
    a. Blood stream.
    b. Local spread (osteomyelitis p. 158).
    c. As a result of wound of the joint.
2. Trauma—synovitis. It could be direct violence or a dislocation possibly associated with a fracture.

Clinical features
1. The local tissues are swollen, painful and warm (local response p. 9).
2. There is an effusion in the joint.
3. There is limitation of movement caused by muscle spasm.
4. With an infection the patient has a general malaise and pyrexia (general response p. 10).

Treatment

Synovitis
1. Immobilisation of joint
2. Firm bandaging to assist reabsorption of fluid.
3. Aspiration may help reabsorption.
4. Eventual gradual mobilisation.

Acute infection
1. Immobilisation of joint.
2. Antibiotics.
3. Aspiration to identify organisms.
4. Eventual gradual mobilisation.

CHRONIC ARTHRITIS
Rheumatoid and osteoarthritis are the main types.

Rheumatoid arthritis
A general systemic disease of unknown aetiology, which involves the joints, mainly of the limbs, especially the hands and feet. There is an inflammation of the capsule and synovial membrane. The synovial membrane pushes into the joint space and may become attached to the articular cartilage. Later with healing, fibrosis in the capsule and synovial membrane can cause gross distortion of the joints.

Clinical features
1. Systemically the patient is unwell with malaise, pyrexia and tachycardia.
2. Locally the joints are painful and swollen.

Treatment
1. Initially it is medical with aspirin and other anti inflammatory drugs and physiotherapy. Occasionally steroids are used.
2. Surgery is now frequently used in:
    a. Synovectomy (excision of the excess synovial membrane) in the early stages.
    b. In the later stages surgery is used to correct deformities and replace destroyed joints with artificial ones.

Osteoarthritis
A disease mainly of later life and is a local condition in contrast to rheumatoid arthritis. The articular cartilage degenerates and eventually bone articulates with bone. There is proliferation of the synovial membrane into the joint, but not as a result of inflammation (unlike rheumatoid arthritis). A past history of injury to the joint is not infrequent.

Clinical features
1. Pain and stiffness in the joint.
2. Limitation of movement.

Treatment
1. Conservative measures consist of physiotherapy and exercises and if necessary weight reduction.
2. More of these joints are now being treated if severe enough by their replacement by artificial joints, especially the hip and knee joints.

Special conditions

CONGENITAL DISLOCATION OF THE HIP
The child is born with the hip dislocated. Clinically one leg is shorter than the other and the buttocks are asymmetrical. It may be bilateral. The slightest suspicion requires careful clinical assessment and the child must be X-rayed, for early treatment gives very good results.

Treatment is by reduction and splinting for some months. If not detected early, it becomes much more difficult to treat and requires surgery.

PERTHES' DISEASE (Pseudo-coxalgia)
Children develop degeneration and necrosis of the bone in the femoral head, which eventually collapses with distortion of the surface unless it is diagnosed and treated early. The cause is unknown.

Clinically, there is pain and limitation of movement and X-ray gives the diagnosis.

Treatment is rest and non-weight-bearing until healing is complete. Osteoarthritis in later life follows, if there is any distortion.

SLIPPED EPIPHYSIS
In adolescence the head of the femur can become displaced on the neck of the bone at the epiphyseal plate. The cause of the slip is unknown. There is pain and limitation of movement.

Treatment is designed to stop further displacement by bed rest and often internal fixation of the head.

TORN SEMILUNAR CARTILAGE
The two semilunar cartilages lie between the articular surfaces of the femur and tibia. A violent twist to the knee may cause the femoral condyle to crush through the medial cartilage splitting it. This interferes with movement and the knee joint may 'lock' in flexion.

Treatment is surgical removal of the cartilage.

TALIPES EQUINO VARUS (club foot)
The child is born with a normal foot grossly twisted out of shape at the joints.

Treatment is gentle manipulation to the normal shape and maintenance if necessary with strapping, or a plaster cast. Very severe cases may require operative correction.

HALLUX VALGUS
Due to ill fitting shoes, the big toes are pushed laterally to the extent of the metacarpal head becoming prominent medially (bunion). The exposed head is easily injured and becomes very painful.

Treatment
1. The best is prevention with proper shoes.
2. Surgical correction is needed for the established case.

33 Dislocation

Dislocation is a complete derangement of a joint.

Aetiology

1. *Trauma.* If associated with a fracture, it is a fracture dislocation.
2. *Congenital.* Some children are born with a dislocation, e.g. of the hip (p. 172).
3. *Pathological.* Due to destruction of the bone, e.g. tuberculosis of spine (p. 159).

Clinical features

1. *Deformity* at the joint—there is often a gap where a bone is normally felt.
2. *Loss of movement*—The muscles cannot act properly on the bones.
3. *Swelling*—This may be severe in traumatic cases and may mask the deformity.
4. *Pain* is present and also severe in traumatic cases.

Treatment

1. By gentle manipulation the joint surfaces are realigned. This often requires general anaesthesia to relax the muscles.
2. Open operation may be necessary, especially where soft tissues have become interposed.
3. The joint is supported with strapping, with a plaster cast, e.g. hip, to allow the stretched ligaments to recover.
4. Physiotherapy is commenced immediately to maintain the muscles and active exercises may be started early to encourage full movement, especially with the shoulder joint.

Fracture dislocation

Commonest in the upper limb. It may make the treatment of the dislocation much more difficult. Generally the fracture is reduced first and then the dislocation.

Sprains

Less injury than a dislocation. The ligaments around a joint are torn. There is pain and swelling. Treatment is support with strapping or firm bandages to allow the ligaments to heal. If very severe, immobilisation in a plaster cast may be required.

Shoulder joint

The shallow glenoid cavity of the scapula makes dislocation fairly common and is usually caused by a fall on the outstretched arm. Reduction is usually easy. The joint is immobilised in a sling for three weeks, except in the elderly where active exercises are encouraged early.

Recurrent dislocation of the shoulder is not uncommon and surgery may be required to cure it.

Elbow joint

A fall on the hand may dislocate the elbow posteriorly. Reduction is followed by restriction of movement in a sling or a plaster cast for three weeks to allow healing of the capsule.

Metacarpophalangeal and interphalangeal joints

Dislocation is caused by hyper-extension. The joint is gently reduced by manipulation but open operation may be required to take soft tissues out of the way.

Hip joint

Great force is required and is commonly the result of a car accident. As the person is seated, a blow on the knee from the dash board is transmitted along the femur and drives the head posteriorly out of the acetabulum where it is shallowest.

Treatment is reduction under general anaesthesia and a plaster cast for six weeks, or bed rest with light traction to rest the joint and allow the ligaments to heal.

Dislocation of the knee and lower limbs are very infrequent, apart from the ankle where it is associated with fracture dislocation (Pott's fracture, p. 169).

34 Muscles, tendons and bursae

Muscle rupture
Occasionally with violent exercise or sudden muscle spasm a muscle or the tendon of it will rupture.

THIGH MUSCLE (RECTUS FEMORIS) AND TENDON
It may rupture with a badly timed kick at football (the sudden jerk tears it).

A gap is seen and can be felt anteriorly in the mid thigh and extension of the knee is greatly weakened. It is treated by immobilisation in a plaster cast for six weeks.

In the elderly patient, it is rather the muscle tendon or the patella ligament that ruptures.

A gap is seen and felt above or below the patella. Extension at the knee is lost.

Treatment is operative repair.

TENDON ACHILLES
With violent exercise, the tendon is torn from the heel bone, often when playing squash. It is commonest in early middle age.

Clinical features
1. A gap is seen and felt above the heel.
2. The patient cannot stand on 'tiptoe'.

Treatment
Surgical repair is necessary, followed by a plaster cast for six weeks.

TENNIS ELBOW
A painful condition, probably associated with the tearing of some muscle fibres at the elbow.

Clinical features
1. Acute pain at the lateral aspect of the elbow on pronation, and gripping of the hand.
2. The site is very tender to palpation.

Treatment
1. Local injection of cortisone may relieve it.
2. Persistent cases are best treated with a sling. It is a self resolving condition given time.

ACUTE TENOSYNOVITIS
Inflammation of a tendon sheath usually of the extensor muscles at the wrist.

Aetiology
It is commonly due to unaccustomed repetitive exercise, e.g. the return to factory work after a vacation.

Clinical features
Pain over the tendon on movement and it may even 'creak'.

Treatment
It is treated by rest and it may require a plaster cast to the forearm and hand.

ACUTE SUPPURATIVE TENOSYNOVITIS
Infection of the tendon sheaths is now uncommon due to antibiotics. It follows a wound or local spread of infection (p. 10).

TRIGGER FINGER
The flexor tendon sheath of a finger becomes thickened and constricted. The tendon as it moves in the sheath, snaps through the constriction and the finger jerks into flexion or extension.

Treatment is the surgical splitting of the constriction in the sheath.

GANGLION
Consists of a cyst lined by synovial membrane and connected to a synovial tendon sheath or a joint. It contains thick clear jelly.

Treatment is to try to burst them by pressure, but more certain is surgical excision.

DUPUYTREN'S CONTRACTURE
The fascia in the palm which runs into the base of the fingers becomes invaded by fibroblasts. The resultant fibrous tissue contracts, shortening the fascia. The cause is unknown, but is partly congenital.

Clinical features
1. Irregular thickening of the fascia can be seen and felt.
2. Flexion contractures of the fingers, especially the third, fourth and fifth.

Treatment
Surgical excision of the fibrous tissue.

TRAUMATIC DIVISION OF TENDONS
Commonly it is the tendons of the hand or wrist that are cut, with subsequent loss of movement.

Treatment
If the wound is clean and the damage minimal, the tendons are sutured immediately, if not, it is carried out after three weeks, after the wound has healed. Prolonged physiotherapy will be required to overcome the adhesions, which often form and limit movement. Tendon grafting may be required for badly damaged finger tendons, less important tendons being sacrificed to act as the grafts.

Bursa

A bursa is a closed synovial sac situated over joints to allow the skin to move with the joint movement.

BURSITIS
Inflammation of a bursa, which fills with fluid. Usually due to repeated slight trauma, but can be infection. Suppurative bursitis is treated with antibiotics and possible drainage.

ACROMIAL BURSITIS
Inflammation of the bursa lying above the humeral head and below the acromion. Causes severe pain in the shoulder and marked limitation of movement.

Treatment
Treatment is physiotherapy assisted by local injection of cortisone.

PREPATELLAR BURSITIS (Housemaids knee)
The bursa anterior to the patella becomes inflamed by repeated kneeling.

Treatment
Stop kneeling! Aspiration and a pressure bandage may be successful, but if not surgical excision.

Finger and hand infections

Most hand and finger infections are the result of a minor penetrating injury, e.g. thorn prick. The common organism is staphylococcus.

PARONYCHIA
An infection at the root of the nail in the fold. It spreads beneath the root and may become an abscess.

Treatment
Early antibiotics may cure it. An abscess will require surgical drainage.

CHRONIC PARONYCHIA
Commonly a fungal infection. Found where the hands are often damp—washing up without gloves.

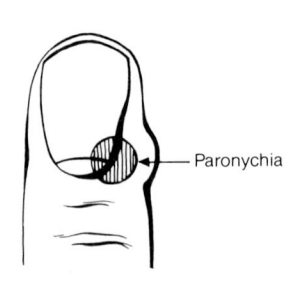

Figure 34.1 Paronychia

MUSCLES, TENDONS AND BURSAE 179

Treatment
Treatment is of the fungus.

PULP INFECTION (Whitlow)
The pulp of the terminal phalanx is divided by fibrous tissue into numerous compartments imprisons any infection. A high tension quickly builds up and the pressure created can thrombose the artery and lead to necrosis of the distal bone. The increased tension makes this a most painful condition.

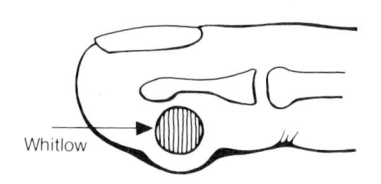

Figure 34.2 Pulp infection (Whitlow)

Treatment
Antibiotics and if not quickly settled, incision and drainage.

WEB SPACE INFECTIONS
These are in the loose web tissue between the fingers. If incision and drainage is required, it is carried out through the dorsum of the hand.

PALMAR INFECTION
The palm is divided into compartments by fibrous tissue. Infection is limited by the fibrous tissue. There is a danger of involvement of the tendons.

Treatment is antibiotics with early incision and drainage.

SUBUNGUAL HAEMATOMA
A haemorrhage under a nail the result of a blow. It is extremely painful. Treatment is to drill a hole in the nail, which immediately gives relief.

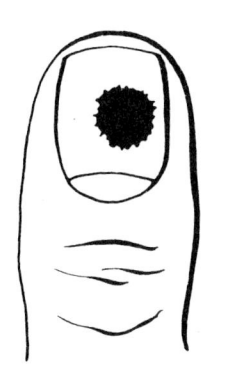

Figure 34.3 Subungual haematoma

Feet

The anatomy of the feet resembles that of the hand. Infections, although less common, follow a similar pattern and are treated in the same way.

INGROWING TOE NAIL
Seen mainly in the adolescent where the growth of the feet is outstripping the size of shoe or stocking. The feet become cramped and the big toe is squeezed laterally against the second toe, resulting in the lateral nail fold of the big toe being pushed over the nail. Chronic infection (paronychia) develops and the nail is further buried eventually in granulation tissue.

Treatment
1. Excise the overhanging nail fold and a wedge of nail bed to clear the infection.
2. Ensure there is ample room in shoes and stockings in future.

ONYCHOGRYPHOSIS
Often as a result of an injury—the nail as well as growing lengthwise, grows in thickness. Develops also in the elderly, possibly the result of a fungal infection.

Treatment
1. Regular chiropody will keep it in check.
2. Surgical excision of the nail and nail bed is preferred by many patients.

PLANTAR WARTS
Found mainly in the young. It is a viral infection frequently passed in swimming pools. Pressure from walking causes it to 'grow' into the epidermis and become painful.

Treatment
Local application of a caustic-glacial acetic acid destroys it.

35 Kidney

Each kidney lies on the posterior abdominal wall protected by the lower ribs. Under a thin fibrous *capsule* lies the *cortex* containing the glomeruli and deeper is the *medulla* formed by the tubules which open on the medullary *papillae* which project into the pelvis forming the *calyces*. The calyces join together forming the *pelvis* which is continuous with the ureter.

The *ureters* run down the posterior abdominal wall into the pelvis, where they open into the base of the bladder. The calyces, pelvis and ureter are formed of smooth muscle lined by transitional cell epithelium. This smooth muscle passes the urine by *peristalsis* from the pelvis of the kidney to the bladder.

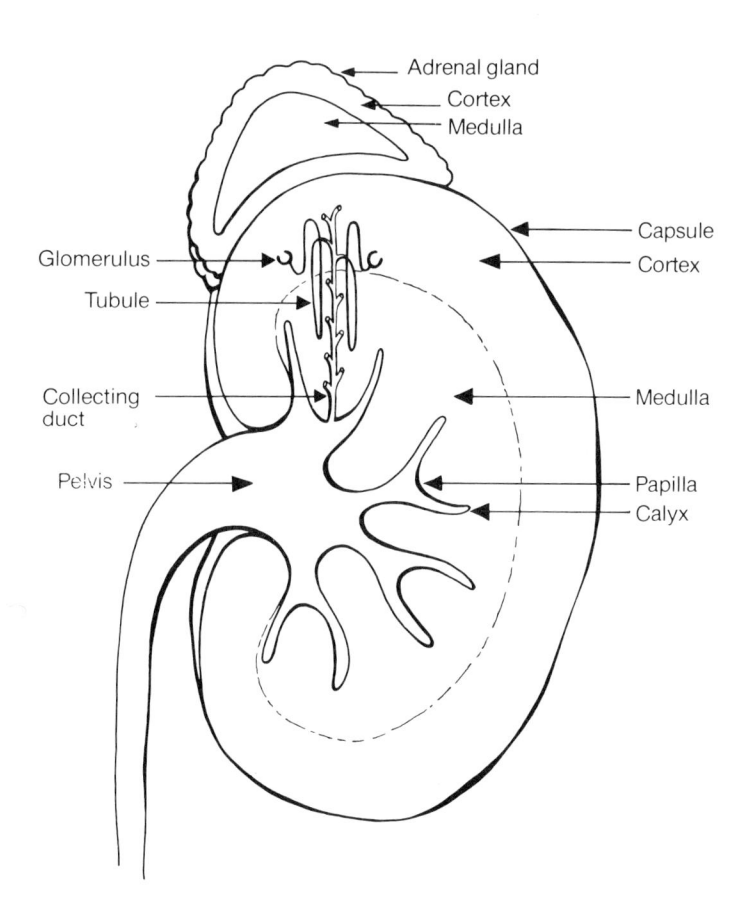

Figure 35.1
Kidney

ESSENTIAL SURGERY FOR NURSES 182

Special investigations of the urinary tract

INTRAVENOUS PYELOGRAM (i.v.p.)
The urinary tract is outlined by an intravenous dye, which becomes concentrated in the urine by the kidney and becomes visible on X-ray; the pelvis of the kidney, ureter and bladder being outlined.

RETROGRADE PYELOGRAM
Through a cystoscope, thin ureteric catheters are passed into the kidney pelvis. Urine samples may be taken and the pelvis may be outlined on X-ray by injected dye.

ARTERIOGRAPHY
Dye injected into the aorta passes into the blood vessels of the kidney which can be outlined on X-ray, and any abnormal distribution seen, as is often present in malignant disease.

SCANNING
Some radioactive chemicals, when injected, are concentrated in the kidney. Special instruments measure the activity and produce on paper a map of the kidney, which will show any areas of poor function, e.g. cyst or tumour.

CYSTOSCOPY
The cystoscope allows direct viewing of the interior of the bladder and the passage of ureteric catheters.

Rupture of the kidney

The result of a severe blow to the loin. The injury can range from a small tear to a complete split.

Clinical features
1. There may be a large swelling in the loin.
2. Haematuria is usual.
3. The patient may be shocked from blood loss.

Treatment
1. Conservative—blood transfusion—may be massive to combat shock.
2. Emergency intravenous pyelogram to confirm the other kidney.
3. Surgery—exploration—if bleeding does not stop.
   A small tear may be repaired but most require nephrectomy.

Congenital conditions

SOLITARY KIDNEY
About 1 in 2000 persons is born with only one kidney and it is usually of no significance for the only one is twice the normal size.

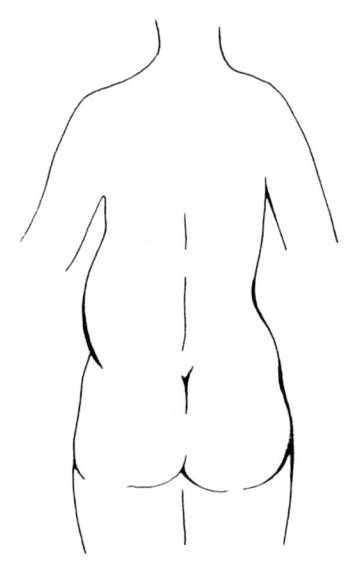

Figure 35.2
Loin swelling (ruptured kidney)

POLYCYSTIC DISEASE

This is a hereditary disease. Kidneys are filled with cysts which slowly enlarge. They press on the adjacent renal tissue and gradually destroy it. The patient eventually develops renal failure. It presents usually after the age of 30.

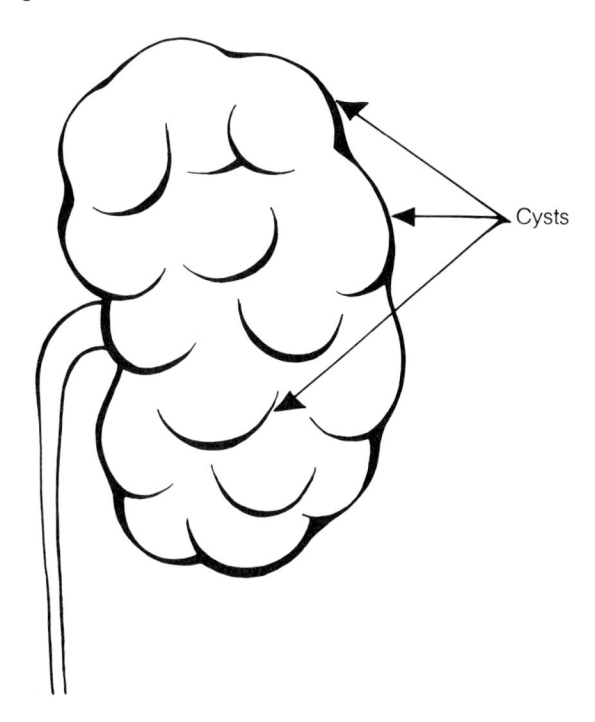

Figure 35.3 Polycystic kidney

Clinical features
1. Aching pain in the loins, associated with large palpable kidneys.
2. Most develop hypertension.
3. Haematuria.
4. i.v.p. confirms the disease.

Treatment

Medical
1. Diet (low protein) to delay renal failure.
2. Renal dialysis (eventually) with artificial kidney.

Surgery
1. Puncturing the cysts relieves the pain (Rovsings operation).
2. When the kidneys fail—patients are candidates for renal dialysis and transplant.

RENAL CYSTS

Isolated renal cysts unassociated with polycystic disease may develop. Most cause no symptoms and are not treated. A few become very large and are excised.

Hydronephrosis

An obstruction to the outlet of the urine, which causes dilatation of the calyces and pelvis of the kidney. The renal tissue becomes stretched over the dilation and is slowly destroyed. If the ureter is involved and is dilated hydro-ureter results.

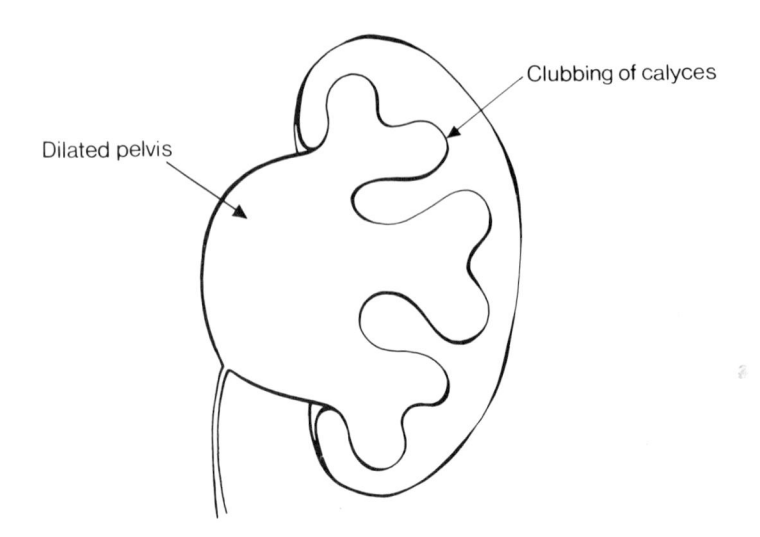

Figure 35.4
Congenital hydronephrosis

Aetiology

Acquired
1. Blockage in the lumen of the pelvis or ureter, by e.g. calculus, tumour.
2. Narrowing in the wall of the ureter, e.g. stricture from injury, infection, tuberculosis.
3. Pressure from without on the ureter—e.g. carcinoma of the cervix, metastatic lymph glands.
4. Back pressure from the bladder due to urethral obstruction, resulting in bilateral hydroureters and hydronephrosis (p. 199).

Congenital
Born with incoordination of the muscle fibres at the pelvi-ureteric junction, and so the peristaltic wave has difficulty passing over the junction (p. 181).

Clinical features
1. Intermittent pain in the loin.
2. Large swelling in the loin.
3. X-rays confirm the diagnosis.

Complication
1. Gradual destruction of the renal parenchyma by the back pressure.
2. Infection which is very liable to become severe due to the poor drainage—pyonephrosis (p. 185).

Treatment
1. Remove the cause, e.g. calculus.
2. Congenital blockage requires a plastic repair to bypass the junction.
3. If the kidney is badly damaged then nephrectomy.

Pyelonephritis

Infection of the parenchyma and pelvis of the kidney.

Acute
The infection may be blood-borne, but most spread from the bladder via the ureter. It is more frequent in females, especially in early marriage or pregnancy. The commonest organism is *E. coli*.

Clinical features
1. Pain and tenderness over the kidney.
2. Severe pyrexia and general systemic response (p. 10).
3. Frequency of micturition with dysuria.
4. Leucocytes (pus cells) and bacteria in the urine.

Treatment
1. High fluid intake.
2. Antibiotics, Ampicillin 1 to 2 g/day, Co-trimoxazole (Septrin 4 to 6 tablets/day) until the urine is sterile.

Chronic
The result of continuing infection or repeated re-infections. The kidneys are gradually destroyed.

Clinical features
1. Repeated attacks of acute pyelonephritis.
2. There may be none except deteriorating health and eventually impending renal failure.

Treatment
1. Remove all predisposing factors such as calculi or urinary stasis.
2. Long term antibiotics.

Pyonephrosis

The pelvis of the kidney is filled with pus. It is the result of an infection in hydronephrosis (p. 184), but can follow acute pyelonephritis.

Clinical features
Similar to acute pyelonephritis.

Treatment
1. Antibiotics may save the kidney.
2. Nephrectomy is usually necessary.

Perinephric abscess

An abscess in the fatty tissue surrounding the kidney, usually the result of spread from an infection in the kidney, e.g. pyonephrosis (p. 185).

Clinical features
1. Systemic and local signs of infection.
2. Very tender and fluctuant loin swelling.

Treatment
Drainage of the abscess, and removal of the cause which may require nephrectomy.

Calculi

Some of the chemicals in the urine become crystals under certain conditions. These may join together to form clumps (calculi or stones). Most form in the kidney and if small can pass into the ureter and on to the bladder. (They also form in the bladder.)

Predisposing factors
1. Infection of urine—E. coli.
2. Hyperparathyroidism—too much calcium in urine (p. 61).
3. Prolonged bed rest, especially with fractures, causes high calcium secretion.
4. Congenital metabolic disease, e.g. gout (increase of uric acid and urates).
5. In many cases, no cause can be found.

Commonest calculi
1. Calcium oxalate (small, nobbly and very dark).
2. Calcium phosphate (large white and smooth) may fill and take the shape of the pelvis and calyces—a staghorn calculus.
3. Calcium urate (brown, smooth and small).
4. Rare—cysteine and xanthine stones—result of congenital metabolic diseases.

Clinical features
1. Most renal calculi, especially if large (staghorn) cause an aching pain in the loin, associated with tenderness.
2. Smaller calculi (oxalate) may try to enter the ureter and block the pelvi-ureteric junction causing severe loin pain—renal colic due to the smooth muscle spasm and the increased intra pelvic pressure.
3. Calculi which have entered the ureter cause ureteric colic—severe pain often starting in the loin and in the line of the ureter radiating into the testes or labia.
4. Haematuria, from the trauma, to the epithelium is often present.
5. Nausea and vomiting may occur, especially with acute colic.

6. Most calculi can be demonstrated by X-ray.
   But some renal calculi cause no symptoms and are found on X-ray by chance.

Complications
1. Damage to the kidney or ureter from local irritation.
2. Hydronephrosis as a result of urinary blockage (p. 184).
3. Infection—the calculus acts as a foreign body . . . favouring infection (p. 9).
4. Renal failure may eventually develop if both kidneys are involved and destroyed.

Treatment

Treatment of the colic
1. Analgesics for the severe pain (morphine 15 mg).
2. Smooth muscle relaxants for the spasm (atropine 0.5 mg Pro-Banthine 15 to 30 mg).
3. All possible predisposing factors for the calculus are excluded.

Treatment of the calculus
1. Tiny stones may be left and watched for they do little damage and could be voided spontaneously in the urine, which is collected and filtered to confirm the passage of the calculus.
2. Larger stones are removed by incision through the renal pelvis (pyelolithotomy) or if very large (staghorn) through the kidney itself (nephrolithotomy).

URETERIC CALCULI
1. Small stones moving down the ureter are left alone to be passed in the urine—all of which is filtered to find the stone and confirm its passing.
2. Stones that stick and cause symptoms and damage are removed by surgery—uretero-lithotomy. If the stone is near the bladder it may be removed via a cystoscopy using a special wire basket to hook it out of the ureter (Dormia stone catcher).

Tumours

CHILDREN
Wilms tumour (nephroblastoma)—A tumour of high malignancy arising from residual embryonic cells.
   All develop in children, usually in the first four years. They metastasise early to the lungs.

Clinical features
1. Progressive swelling in the loin.
2. Haematuria.
3. Deteriorating general health in the child.

Treatment
Nephrectomy followed by radiotherapy or cytotoxics.

ADULTS
Benign tumours of the kidney are very uncommon.

Carcinoma of the renal parenchyma (hypernephroma)
This tumour arises from the tubules. It can become very large before clinical features develop. It metastasises to the lung and bone by spreading into the renal vein, where malignant cells break off and become emboli (p. 18).

Clinical features
1. Aching in loin with a palpable swelling.
2. Haematuria.
3. Progressive ill health with anaemia.
4. Very occasionally polycythaemia and pyrexia.
5. Metastases in lung or bone may be the first presentation.

Treatment
1. Nephrectomy if possible.
2. Radiotherapy may be used for palliation.

Carcinoma of the renal pelvis
Arises from the transitional cell epithelium. It spreads early down the lumen of the ureter by shed cells becoming implanted on the ureteric or bladder epithelium.

Clinical features
1. Haematuria.
2. The kidney may be palpably enlarged.
3. May cause symptoms of hydronephrosis, by blockage of the urinary flow.
4. May present as a bladder tumour (p. 194).

Treatment
1. Kidney and ureter are removed because of the danger that cells may have become implanted in the ureteric mucosa (nephroureterectomy).

It may start as a premalignant papilloma which is treated in the same way.

Anuria

Complete stoppage of urine excretion.

Aetiology
1. Pre-renal: With very low blood pressure (shock)—there is not enough filtration pressure.

2. Renal: kidney destruction, e.g. injury, overwhelming infection, tubular necrosis can develop from prolonged shock.
3. Post renal: blockage of ureters by, e.g. stones, accidental ligation at pelvic operations.

Clinical features
1. No urine is voided and there is none in the bladder with catheterisation.
2. There is a rise in blood urea after 24 hours.

Treatment
Pre-renal
The cause is removed and fluid intake and electrolytes carefully monitored until recovery.

Renal
Again, if acute, requires careful fluid and electrolyte monitoring, for the body cannot adjust them. Patient may require renal dialysis and renal transplant.

Post renal
1. The cause is removed, or if not possible.
2. Ureteric catheters are passed, which may bypass the obstruction and act as drains.
3. If neither is possible, then draining one kidney (nephrostomy, p. 195) or one ureter (ureterostomy, p. 195) will relieve the emergency.
4. The cause is removed later.

RENAL TRANSPLANT

Where their kidneys have failed, patients may receive kidney grafts (transplants). Prior to the transplant, the blood group of the patient (recipient) is matched very carefully to the blood group of the donor in order to minimise the effect of antibody response by the patient to the foreign kidney.

SOURCE
1. A close relative with similar blood grouping may donate one kidney. This has become uncommon.
2. Healthy kidneys removed immediately after death. Usually the donors are victims of accidents, brain tumours (p. 148).

OPERATION
The renal vessels are anastomosed to the iliac vessels. The kidney lies in the iliac fossa and the ureter is inserted through the bladder wall.

REJECTION
The antibody response to the foreign kidney, which would destroy it, is suppressed with steroids and immunosuppresant drugs (e.g. imuran).

Adrenal glands

Endocrine glands lying above the kidney, which are under the control of the anterior pituitary (ACTH). They have two distinct parts, cortex and medulla (see Fig. 35.1).

CORTEX
This secretes
1. Hormones controlling metabolism.
2. Hormones controlling the salt (sodium and potassium) and water balance of the body.
3. Sex hormones, both male and female in each person.

MEDULLA
This secretes adrenalin and noradrenalin, which mainly constrict and raise the blood pressure (large quantities produced in shock causing sweating, vaso constriction and tachycardia (p. 26). Hypoglycaemia (low blood sugar) is also a stimulant to secretion.

TUMOURS

Cortical tumour
These may be simple adenomas or malignant carcinomas. They can produce bizarre symptoms from excess hormone production.

Excess metabolic hormones cause moon face, increased weight and atrophy of muscle and skin. Cushing's Syndrome (may also be due to excessive stimulation by a pituitary tumour (p. 150)).

Excess sex hormones causes in females atrophy of breasts, amenorrhoea, facial hair (bearded lady).

Medullary tumours

Neuroblastoma
Rare malignant tumour in children mostly before the age of five years.

Clinical features are similar to Wilm's tumour (p. 187).

Treatment. Removal if possible, followed by radiotherapy.

Phaechromocytoma
An uncommon benign tumour in the adult.

Clinical features are of intermittent or continuous hypertension, due to excessive production of adrenalin.

Treatment. Adrenalectomy.

36 Bladder

The bladder, when empty, lies in the pelvis behind the symphysis pubis, partly covered by peritoneum. It is lined by transitional epithelium and has a thick muscle coat named the detrusor muscle. The ureters enter the base forming a triangular area with the urethral opening called the trigone.

During micturition the detrusor muscle contracts and the urethral sphincter relaxes.

The normal adult bladder capacity is 300 to 400 ml.

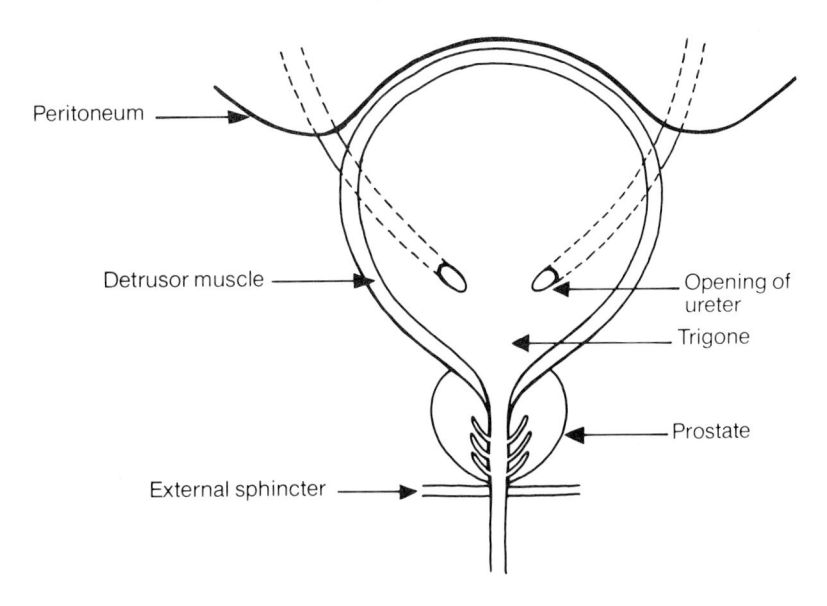

Figure 36.1
Bladder

Rupture

The bladder may be ruptured when full by a severe blow to the abdomen, e.g. kick or be pierced by the bones of a fractured pelvis.

The urine leak may be into the surrounding tissues (extraperitoneal) or into the peritoneal cavity (intraperitoneal).

Clinical features
1. Intense desire to micturate, but the patient can pass only a few drops of blood stained urine.
2. Shock and severe hypogastric pain.
3. Persistently empty bladder clinically and on catheterisation (sometimes a little blood in or on the catheter).
4. Signs of local inflammation or developing peritonitis.

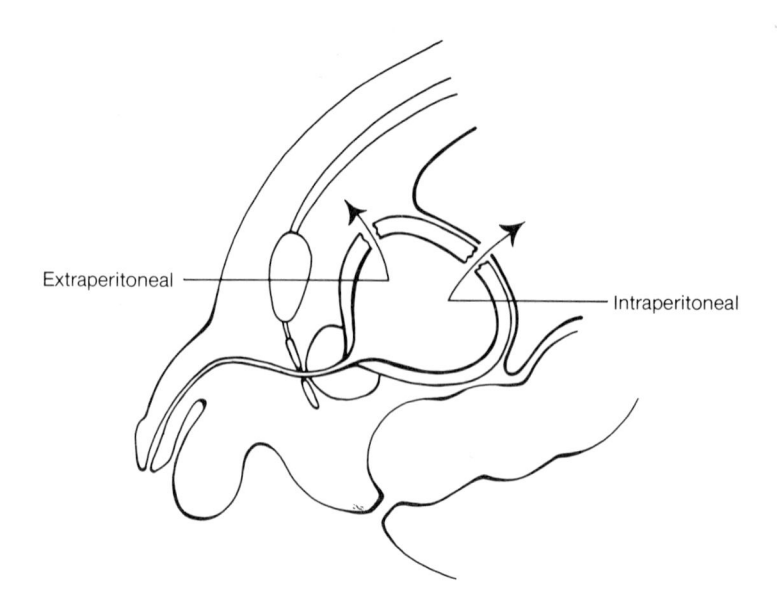

Figure 36.2
Rupture of bladder

Treatment
Immediate surgical repair.

Cystitis

Inflammation of the bladder which may be acute or chronic. It is caused most often by an infection with *E. coli*.

ROUTES OF INFECTION
1. The commonest route of infection is from the urethra and the short female urethra makes cystitis much commoner in females.
2. Infection may pass in the urine to the bladder from an infected kidney.
3. Spread of inflammation locally from another organ may involve the bladder, e.g. appendicitis, Crohn's disease (p. 111).
4. In the male, the prostate is a source of infection (p. 197).

PREDISPOSING FACTORS
1. A foreign body, which causes irritation (e.g. calculus, tumour, faeces from a bowel fistula).
2. Surgical instrumentation causes trauma and introduces infection.
3. Chronic retention of urine (stasis of urine) allows bacteria to multiply.
4. Sexual intercourse. This is a common factor in the female but the reasons are not fully understood.

ACUTE CYSTITIS

Clinical features
1. Frequency of micturition, both diurnal and nocturnal (caused by the irritation of the epithelium.)

2. Dysuria (painful micturition) as the inflamed epithelium is squeezed. It may be suprapubic or perineal.
3. Urgency (intense desire to micturate)—may lead to incontinence.
4. Haematuria—blood in urine from the epithelium bleeding.

Investigation
Mid stream urine specimens of urine are examined and cultured. The first urine (EMU) voided in the morning is examined and cultured for tuberculosis if it is suspected. The bacilli tend to be concentrated in this specimen and more easily found. If recurrent, IVP and cystoscopy to exclude calculi and other causes.

Treatment
1. Remove any predisposing factors, e.g. calculi.
2. Antibiotics (Ampicillin 1 g/day, Co-trimoxazole 4 tablets/day).
3. A high fluid intake causes a diuresis, washing out the bacteria and preventing them multiplying.

CHRONIC CYSTITIS
Continuing or recurrent attacks of cystitis.

Aetiology
1. The presence of a predisposing factor, e.g. tumour.
2. Constant reinfection, e.g. bowel fistula (p. 112).
3. Specific type of infection, e.g. tuberculosis.

Clinical features
Similar to acute cystitis, but prolonged and often less pronounced.

Treatment
1. Full investigation to find any predisposing factor and remove it if possible.
2. High fluid intake dilutes the infection, washing out the bacteria.
3. Antibiotics may help relieve symptoms.
4. Bladder lavage through a catheter with mild antiseptic solution may help in the more difficult case (1:5000 chlorhexidine).

Bladder calculi

They have a similar structure to renal calculi (p. 186).

Aetiology
1. From the kidney (p. 186). Small calculi pass into the bladder and if not voided they will increase in size.
2. Formed in the bladder. Often there is incomplete emptying of urine (residual urine, p. 199) which has become infected.

Clinical features
1. Symptoms of recurrent cystitis, e.g. frequency, haematuria.

2. Pain in the urethra at the end of micturition.
3. Occasional blockage, acute retention
4. Confirmed by X-ray and cystoscopy.

Treatment

Small stones. These are usually crushed (lithopaxy) by a special crushing cystoscope (lithotrite) and the fragments removed by bladder lavage.

Large stones. These require surgery—the bladder is opened (suprapubic lithotomy) and the stones removed.

Tumours

Most arise from the transitional cell epithelium. Aniline dye workers and rubber workers are at special risk due to chemicals used in these industries. Bladder tumours are classified as an industrial disease.

BENIGN
Simple papilloma
These are always potentially malignant.

Clinical features
Painless haematuria.

Treatment
Destruction by diathermy through the cystoscope.

MALIGNANT

Transitional cell carcinoma
May arise from a previous papilloma, or commence as a malignant tumour.

Spread
The tumour may spread superficially before invading the bladder muscle. Having penetrated the bladder it spreads through the perivesical tissues and pelvis. It metastasises late to the lymph glands and distant sites.

Clinical features
1. Haematuria—the tumour is squeezed on micturition.
2. Dysuria, as a result of irritation.
3. Frequency of micturition—diurnal and nocturnal.

Treatment

Superficial tumours (confined to the epithelial surface). Through the cystoscope small tumours are destroyed by electro-coagulation (diathermy).

Superficial large tumours can be removed with a resectoscope. This is a modified cystoscope with a movable electro-cautery knife. This enables the tumour to be cut from the deeper tissues.

Established tumours (invasion of muscle coats). Most are treated by radiotherapy, either by external radiation, or if suitable by local application, e.g. the temporary insertion of radioactive tantullum wire at operation. Some, if small and accessible, can be excised (partial cystectomy). Widespread tumours are palliated by radiotherapy and diathermy.

Total cystectomy has a high operative mortality and requires diversion of the ureters (p. 196) with little long-term benefit over radiotherapy.

Urinary diversions

The urine is diverted to overcome obstruction or disease.

NEPHROSTOMY
A tube can be inserted into the kidney (p. 189) where there is blockage distally either in the case of a solitary kidney, or where both have been blocked.

URETEROSTOMY
May be required for severe bladder disease.

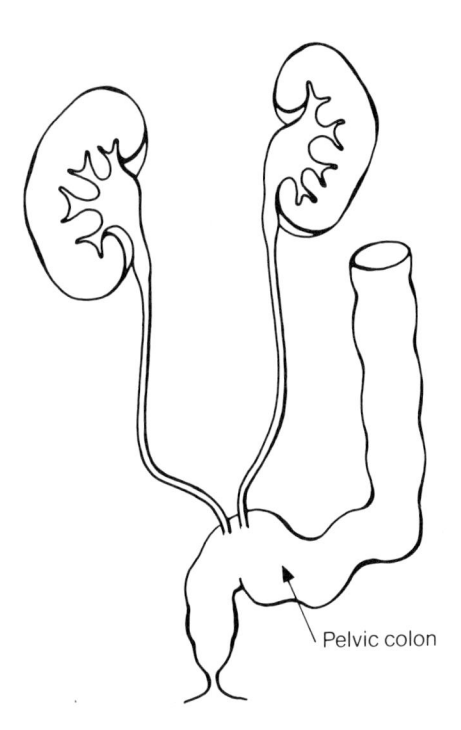

Figure 36.3
Ureterostomy (1)

1. The ureters can be inserted into the pelvic colon. The rectum acts as the reservoir and the patient voids approximately three-hourly. Feaces do not mix with the urine and defaecation is normal.

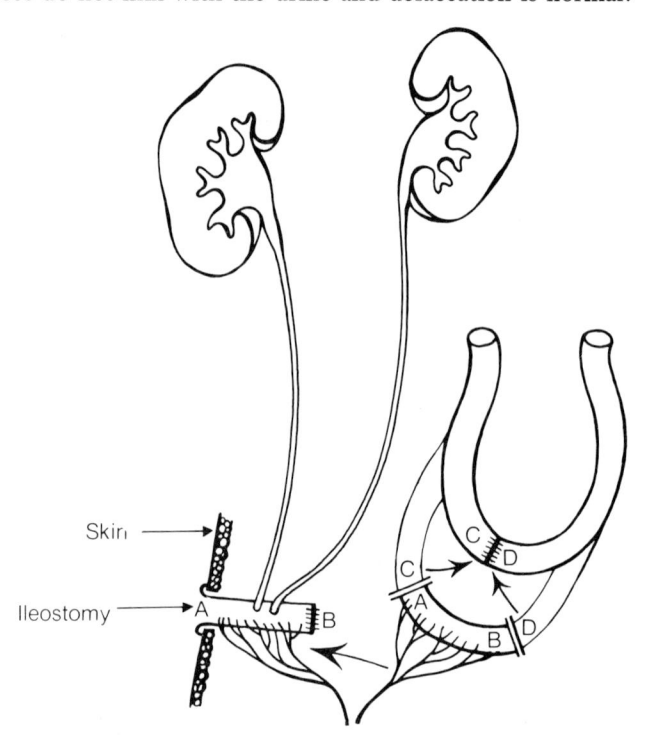

Figure 36.4
Ureterostomy (2)

2. A loop of ileum is isolated with the blood supply intact. One end is closed and the other made into an ileostomy (p. 123). The ureters are inserted into the loop.

SUPRAPUBIC CYSTOSTOMY

A drainage tube is inserted into the bladder suprapubically to bypass urethral obstruction, e.g. stricture. It is usually temporary until the obstruction can be removed.

37 Prostate and urethra

The external sphincter surrounds the urethra below the bladder in the female but in the male the prostate gland intervenes before the sphincter enclosing the urethra. The prostate secretes fluid into the urethra on ejaculation, which nourish the sperm. These enter the prostatic urethra from the vas deferens.

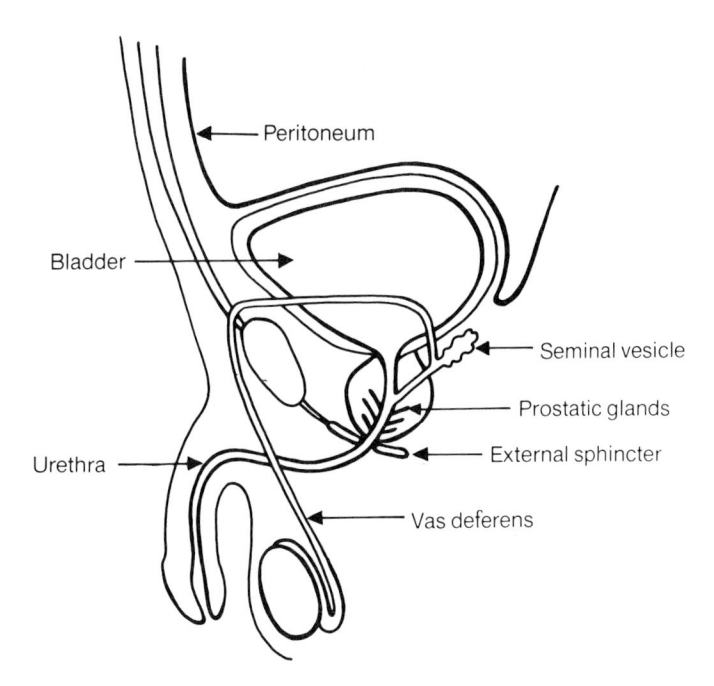

Figure 37.1
Prostate and urethra

The prostate

ACUTE PROSTATITIS
Inflammation of the prostate is due usually to infection. The commonest bacteria is the *E. coli*, but occasionally it is a gonococcal infection.

Clinical features
1. Frequency of micturition is quickly followed by dysuria and haematuria.
2. There is often a general malaise with pyrexia and even rigors.
3. Pain in the perineum and anal canal on defaecation may be present.
4. In very acute cases there is acute retention from spasm of sphincter and oedema.

Treatment
1. Antibiotics (Ampicillin 1 to 2 g/day).
2. Very occasionally catheterisation is required for acute retention.

Complication
The infection may spread to cause cystitis, epididymo-orchitis (p. 206) and even pyelonephritis.

CHRONIC PROSTATITIS
Recurrent infections can gradually destroy the gland which is replaced by fibrous tissue (fibrous prostate), which may narrow the urethra and cause or lead to a stricture (p. 202).

Clinical features
1. Recurrent bouts of acute prostatitis.
2. With time there may be symptoms of a urethral stricture (p. 202).

Treatment
1. Antibiotics will relieve the acute attacks.
2. Stricture formation can be treated by periodic dilatation (bouginage), or a small portion may be removed by resectoscope, i.e. transurethral resection (p. 199).

BENIGN PROSTATIC HYPERTROPHY
Commonly after middle age, due to hormonal changes, the deepest part of the prostate enlarges by forming discrete adenomas. Their enlargement pushes the normal prostatic tissue to the periphery and also narrows the urethra. The enlargement may push up under the bladder base making micturition difficult.

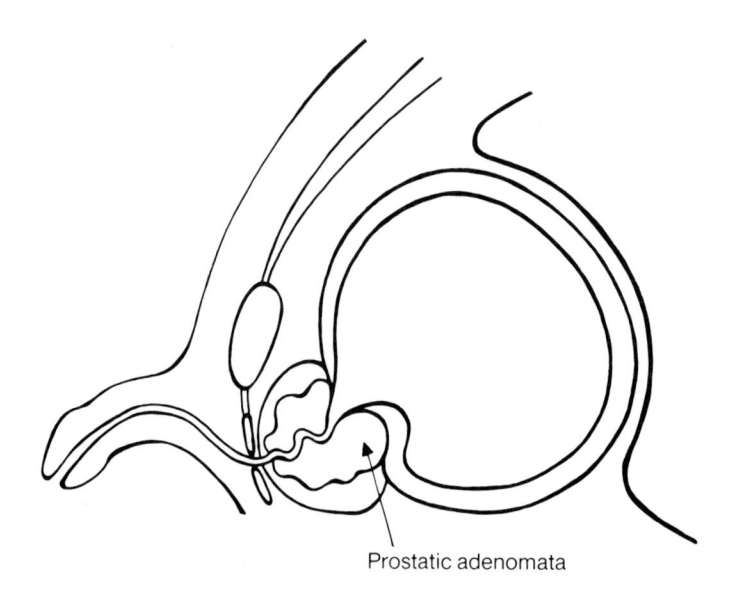

Figure 37.2
Benign prostatic hypertrophy

Prostatic adenomata

The bladder overcomes the resistance by contracting at a higher pressure, but this causes inefficient voiding of smaller quantities and results in a residual urine remaining in the bladder.

Clinical features
1. Frequency (diurnal and nocturnal) as the bladder can only void small quantities.
2. Poor flow results from the narrowed urethra.
3. Haematuria from congestion of bladder base.
4. Acute or chronic retention is common.
5. Hydronephrosis and renal failure if there is severe back pressure (p. 184).

Treatment
1. If the enlargement has not become too great, it can be excised using a modified cystoscope (resectoscope)—transurethral resection (TUR).

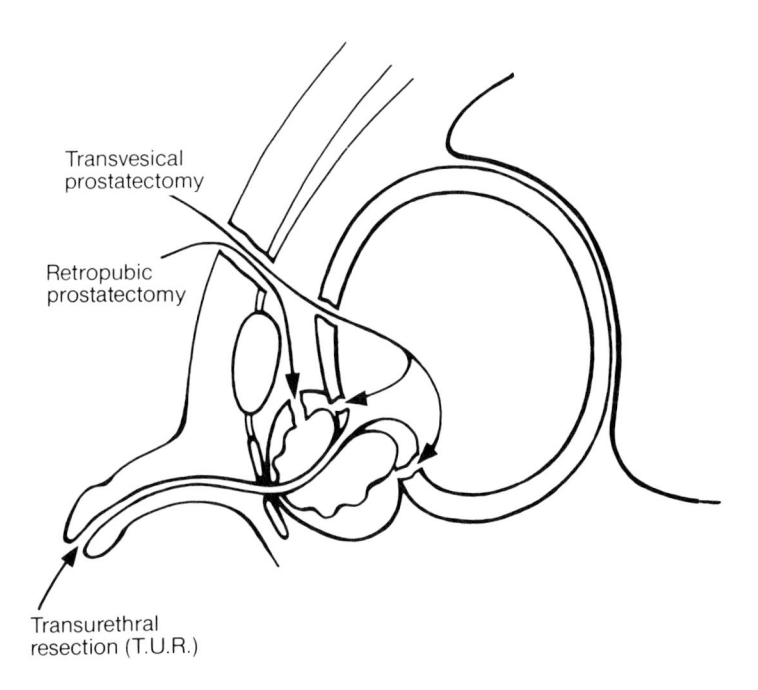

Figure 37.3 Prostatectomy

2. Prostatectomy. Through a suprapubic incision the adenomas only are removed, either by opening the gland directly (retropubic or Millins prostatectomy) or through the bladder (transvesical prostatectomy). Most patients require drainage by a urethral catheter for some days post-operatively.

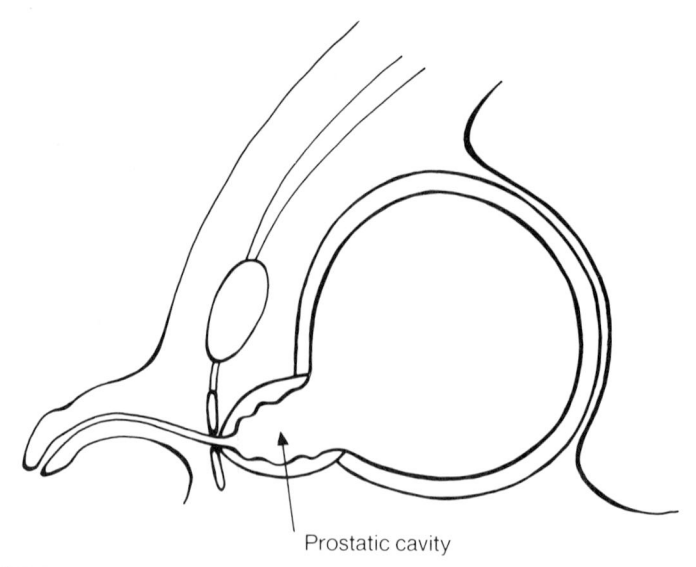

Figure 37.4
Post prostatectomy

Prostatic cavity

CARCINOMA OF PROSTATE

It is a hormone-dependent adenocarcinoma, being stimulated by the male hormone, testosterone, and inhibited by the female hormone oestrogen. Arising in the periphery of the gland it invades not only the rest of the gland but outwards into the pelvis. It metastasises commonly to the pelvic bones and lower vertebrae.

Clinical features
1. These are similar to benign prostatic hypertrophy, but develop quickly in a few months.
2. The hard nodular tumour is felt on rectal examination and can be biopsied per rectum.
3. The blood acid phosphatase level may be raised (it is produced in excess by the malignant cells).
4. Back pain from metastases may be the first symptom.

Treatment (palliative only)
The aim is to reduce male hormone and increase female hormone. So:
1. Remove testes (bilateral orchidectomy).
2. Give female hormones, e.g. stilboestrol 5 mg t.d.s.
3. If the tumour is blocking the urethra, then portions may be removed by the resectoscope (p. 199).
4. New techniques of treatment by radiotherapy are being tested with promising results.

RETENTION OF URINE

Acute retention is the sudden cessation of micturition.

Chronic retention is the result of a progressive obstruction to micturition. The increasing difficulty causes the bladder muscle to hypertrophy, which results in it becoming less efficient, and an increasingly large residual urine develops.

Eventually the bladder is permanently dilated—chronic retention.

Aetiology

Mechanical. There are many physical causes of blockage to the urethra:
1. In the urethral lumen, e.g. calculus.
2. In the wall—uretheral stricture.
3. Pressure on the urethral wall—prostatic hypertrophy, paraphimosis.

Clinical features
1. Progressive slowing of the urinary stream.
2. Worsening frequency of micturition and nocturia due to the inefficient emptying.
3. Abdominal distension from the dilated bladder.

Treatment
1. Catheterisation, which may have to be preceded by bouginage. If unsuccessful, suprapubic drainage may be temporarily necessary.
2. Investigation and treatment of the cause.

Urethra

RUPTURE OF THE URETHRA

The rupture can be complete or incomplete.

Aetiology
1. Fractured pelvis where the urethra is pulled apart by the separation of the bones (intrapelvic).
2. A blow to the perineum, which splits the urethra (bulbous) against the pubis.

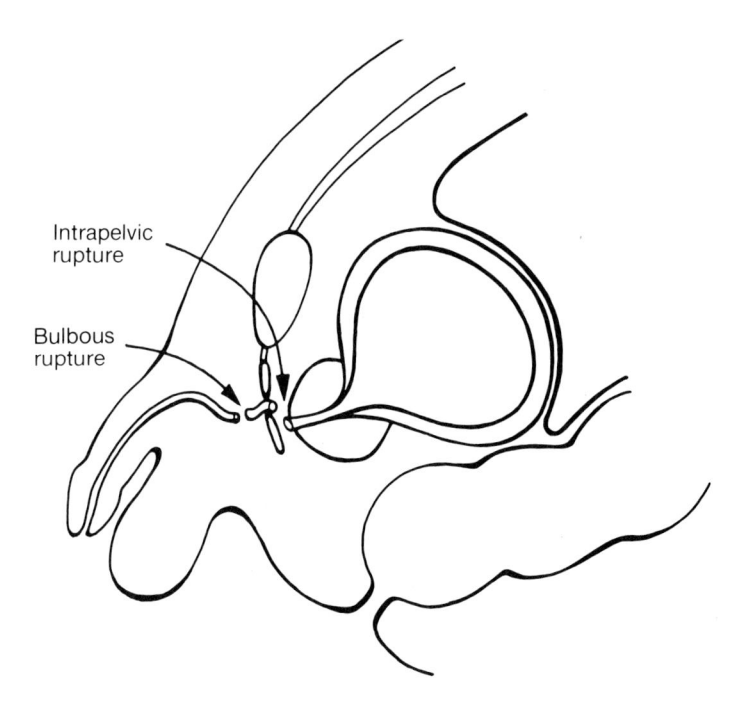

Figure 37.5
Rupture of urethra

Clinical features
1. History of injury with fractured pelvis or perineal injury.
2. Retention of urine. All attempts at micturition result in the urine extravasating into the pelvic tissue (intrapelvic) or the perineal tissues (bulbous).
Patients suspected of ruptured urethra must not try to micturate.
3. Perineal haematoma—develops in a bulbous rupture.
4. Ill-defined suprapubic swelling.

Treatment
1. All suspected cases are catheterised.
2. With incomplete tears, the catheter will pass, and drainage is continued for one week to allow healing.
3. With a complete tear the catheter will not pass, and open cystostomy and perineal exposure of the rupture may be required. A catheter is left in for two to three weeks to allow healing.
4. Drainage of tissues if extravasation has occurred.

Complications
Stricture of the urethra is a frequent late complication.

URETHRAL STRICTURE
Narrowing of the urethra due mostly to fibrous or scar tissue. The eventual effect is similar to prostatic hypertrophy, being inefficient voiding, and a residual urine.

Aetiology
1. Trauma—rupture of the urethra.
2. Infection, e.g. venereal, prostatis (p. 198).
3. Post-operative—prostatectomy.

Clinical features
1. The urinary flow becomes poor.
2. Frequency of micturition and nocturia.
3. May present as acute or chronic retention.

Treatment
1. Gentle periodical dilatation (bouginage) may be sufficient.
2. Surgical excision and repair may be of value in post traumatic cases.

HYPOSPADIAS
Failure of the distal penile urethra to develop properly results in the urethral opening being situated anywhere on the under surface of the penis.

Treatment
At about four years of age, the defect is bridged by plastic surgery.

PHIMOSIS
Narrowing of the orifice of the prepuce. May be severe enough to cause retention. Can be congenital or the result of infections causing scarring.

PARAPHIMOSIS
The prepuce has been retracted, but cannot be made to return and cover the glans penis. It presents as a grossly oedematous ring behind the glans penis.

Treatment

The treatment for both phimosis and paraphimosis is circumcision.

BALANITIS
Inflammation of the surface of the glans penis. It develops most commonly in cases of phimosis, where hygiene is difficult. Occasionally it is due to a fungal infection. Diabetes is a predisposing factor.

Treatment

Remove any precipitating factor. Circumcision is necessary for a phimosis and allows cleaning of the glans.

PENILE WARTS
They are caused by a virus and are fairly common and often multiply. Most are treated by electro coagulation under anaesthesia.

CARCINOMA OF THE PENIS
It presents as a malignant ulcer of the glans in the uncircumcised. Diagnosis is made by biopsy.

Treatment

Treatment is surgical amputation or radiotherapy.

38 Testes

The testes develop in the abdomen and migrate before birth via the inguinal canal to the scrotum. In doing so they take a tube of peritoneum with them, the distal part of which remains as a closed sac (tunical vaginalis) around the testes, but the proximal portion in the cord atrophies. If the tube remains patent proximally, it may present as a congenital inguinal hernia (p. 98). The migration is necessary for the testes require a lower than body temperature for correct development of spermatogenesis, although hormone production (testosterone) is unaffected.

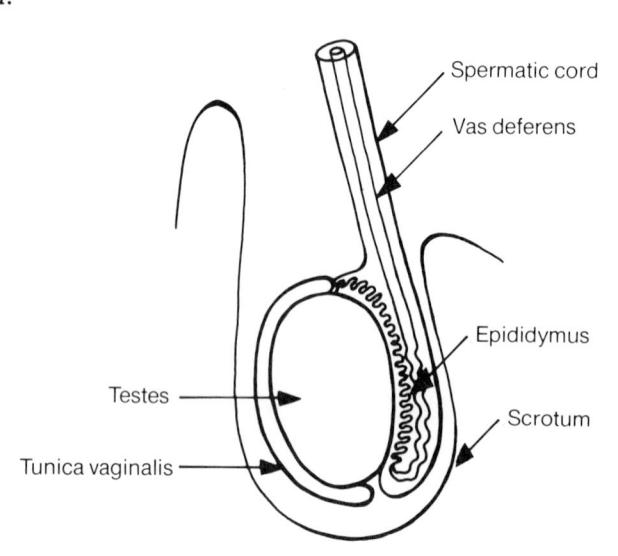

Figure 38.1 Testes

Undescended testes

Occasionally one or both testes do not migrate fully before birth and are usually found in the inguinal region. If left, they will become sterile, certainly by puberty. They are also more liable to injury and to becoming malignant, but this is a relatively small risk.

Treatment
At operation the testes is exposed and placed in the scrotum (orchidopexy). Should the spermatic cord be too short to allow the testes to enter the scrotum, the testes is removed (orchidectomy), provided the other is normal.

But if it is the only testis, it is left, as it is the only source of hormone, the risk of malignancy being accepted.

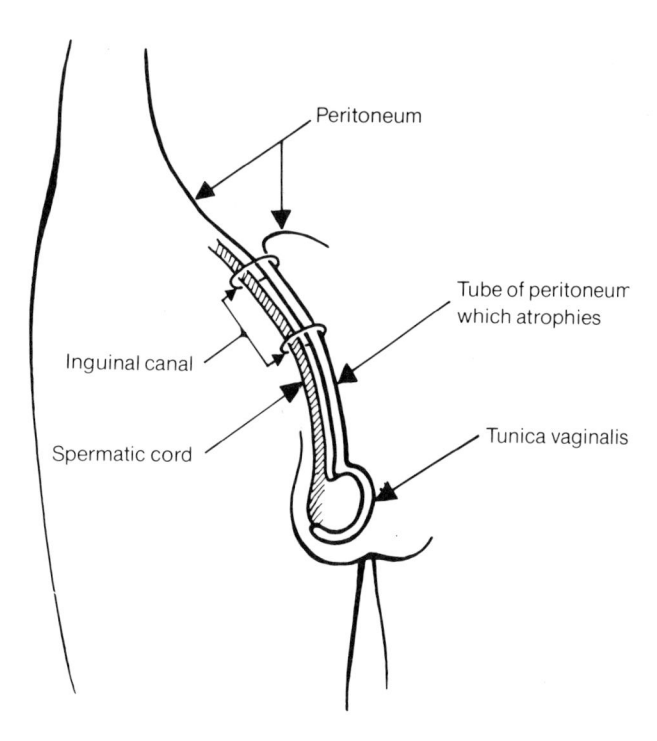

Figure 38.2
Descent of testes

Torsion of testes

The testes twists on the spermatic cord, or in the tunica vaginalis at its junction with the epididymis. The blood supply is interrupted and it becomes gangrenous.

Clinical features
1. Sudden severe pain in testes, associated with marked tenderness and swelling.
2. Oedema and redness of the scrotal skin.

Treatment
1. Emergency surgery, if the testes is dead, orchidectomy.
2. Exploration and fixation of other testis, in case it should twist also, which in effect would castrate the patient.

Epididymitis

Inflammation of the epididymis, usually as a result of a spread of infection from a prostatitis (p. 198) via the vas deferens.

Orchitis

Usually viral (mumps) but may be spread from epididymitis and result in epididymo-orchitis.

Epididymo-orchitis

Clinical features
1. Swollen tender epididymis and testes.
2. Scrotal skin red and oedematous.
3. Pyrexial.

Treatment
1. Rest in bed with a scrotal support.
2. Antibiotics (Ampicillin 2 g/day).

Hydroceles

Filling of the tunica vaginalis around testes with fluid. Can be very large. The cause is usually unknown, but it may follow an epididymitis.

Treatment
1. Tapping of the fluid gives temporary relief.
2. Surgical removal of tunica vaginalis is more satisfactory.

Haematocele

Blood in the tunica vaginalis usually due to trauma.

Treatment
1. Most resolve with time.
2. Evacuate blood through an incision, if it is very large, or becomes infected.

Varicocele

A congenital dilatation or varicosity of the spermatic cord veins of the left testis.

Clinical features
1. It may cause an aching in the left testis and spermatic cord after prolonged standing.
2. It may be associated with a low sperm count.
3. The varicose veins are obvious on standing, but empty when the patient lies down.

Treatment
1. If it is found incidentally and is causing no symptoms, then nothing is done.
2. Where it is causing discomfort, or there is a low sperm count, the veins are ligated.

Tumour of testes

They are comparatively uncommon and most are malignant. Two main groups depending on the type of malignant cells.
1. Seminoma, which arise from the tubules of the testes.
2. Teratoma are thought by some to develop from original embryonic cells which have survived. Both types spread to the aortic lymph glands and the lungs.

Clinical features
Swelling of the testes, which is often very large and painless.

Treatment
1. Orchidectomy, which is followed by
2. Radiotherapy to the aortic lymph nodes.

Male infertility

In about 40 per cent of childless marriages, the husband is found to be subfertile or infertile.

Normal sperm count: 40 to 50 million motile sperm/ml seminal fluid or above.

Oligospermia: less than 20 million sperm/ml seminal fluid.

Azoospermia: no sperm present in the seminal fluid.

Aetiology
1. Non descent of the testes must be corrected well before puberty or it will cause atrophy of the sperm forming cells.
2. Occasional congenital (genetic) defects, i.e. chromosomal abnormalities result in azoospermia and can be identified by examination of the chromosomes in the nuclei of white blood cells.
3. Varicoceles in some patients can cause oligospermia, possibly the increased blood flow raising the testicular temperature.
4. In most patients the cause is unknown.

Treatment
1. Surgical ligation of a varicocele, if present, may improve the count.
2. Where no cause is found, prolonged mild stimulation of the testes with male hormone may improve oligospermia. Mesterolone 100 mg/day for 6 to 12 months.

Vasectomy

An increasingly popular method of contraception, which is used when the parents have the desired number of children. Under local or general anaesthesia a 2 cm, portion of each vas deferens is removed and the cut ends ligated. The testes suffer no ill effects.

Although considered permanent, in special circumstances such as divorce the patient may desire its reversal and the cut ends are reanastomosed. In about 75 per cent of cases this is successful and results in the patient being fertile again.

Index

Abscess, Acute, 10
  Cold, 14
  Diverticular, 121
  Ischio-Rectal, 127
  Pelvic, 95
  Perineal, 127
  Perinephric, 186
  Pilonidal, 5
  Subphrenic, 95
  (See also under organs)
Achalasia, 88
Achondroplasia, 161
Acromegaly, 150
Adenoids, 62
  Hypertrophy of, 64
Adenoma, 17
  of colon, 123
  of pancreas, 136
  of salivary glands, 56
  of thyroid, 60
Adhesions, 96
Adrenals, 190
  Tumours of, 190
Amputations, 41
Aorta, Aneurysm of, 37
  Coarctation of, 85
Aneurysm, 37
  Cerebral, 147
Anuria, 188
Anus, Carcinoma of, 125
  Fissure of, 129
  Perianal haematoma of, 129
  Pruritus ani, 129
Appendicitis, 113
Appendix, 112
  Abscess, 114
Arteriography, Brain, 142
  Kidney, 182
Arthritis, 171
  Acute, 171
  Chronic, 172
  Infective, 171
  Rheumatoid, 172
Atheroma, 37
Avasuclar necrosis, 164

Bacteraemia, 11
Bacteria, 12
  Bacillus coli, 12
  Bacillus tuberculosis, 14
  Clostridium tetani, 12
  Clostridium welchii, 13
  Staphylococcus aureus, 12
  Streptococcus pyogenes, 12
Balanitis, 203

Bile ducts, 138
  Calculi, 140
Bladder, 191
  Calculus, 193
  Carcinoma, 194
  Cystitis, 192
  Papilloma, 194
  Rupture, 191
Blood groups, 32
Blood transfusion, 32
Body scan, 76
Brain, 142
  Abscess, 149
  Death, 147
  Injury, 144
  Scan, 143
  Tumours, 148
Breast, 73
  Abscess, 74
  Carcinoma, 75
  Cyst, 74
  Duct papilloma, 75
  Fibroadenoma, 75
  Fibradenonis, 74
  Mastitis, 73
Burns, 20
  Assessment of, 21
  Classification of, 20
  Fluid replacement in, 22
  Resuscitation in, 22
  Treatment, 23
Bursa, 178
Bursitis, 178

Caecostomy, 129
Calcitonin, 58
Calculi, *(See under organ)*
Carbimazole, 60
Carbuncle, 45
Carcinoma, 18
  Basal cell, 46
  Squamous cell, 46
  (See also under organ)
Cardiac tamponade, 80
Cardiospasm, 88
Celestin tube, 92
Cellulitis, 10
Central venous pressure, 27
Chest injuries, 78
  Open, 78
  Closed, 78
Cholangiogram
  Intravenous, 138
  Percutaneous, 139
Cholangiopancreatography, 139

Cholecystitis, Acute, 139
　Chronic, 140
Cholecytogram, 138
Chondroma, 17, 161
Cimetidine, 89, 105
Circulation, Collateral, 39
Claudication, Intermittent, 39
Club foot, 173
Colic, Biliary, 140
　Renal, 186
　Ureteric, 186
Colon, 120
　Adenoma of, 123
　Carcinoma of, 123
　Colitis ulcerative of, 122
　Megacolon, 121
　Preparation for surgery, 127
Colostomy, 128
Contractures, 21
Coronary artery disease, 86
Crepitations, 80
Crepitus, 79, 164
Crohn's disease (see Regional enteritis), 111
Cushing's syndrome, 190
Cyst, Branchial, 56
　Inclusion dermoids, 45
　Sebaceous, 45
　Thyroglossal, 57
　(See also under organ)

Dermoid cyst, 45
Dextran, 33
Dislocation, 174
　Congenital, 172
　of ankle, 175
　of elbow, 175
　of hand, 175
　of hip, 175
　of shoulder, 175
Diverticulitis, 120
Diverticulosis, 120
Drain, Waterseal, 78
Ductus arteriosus, 85
Dumping syndrome, 109
Duodenum, 103
　Perforation, 107
　Pyloric stenosis, 108
　Ulceration, 105
Dupuytrens contracture, 177

Ear, 67, 70
　Bat, 67
　Carcinoma, 68
　Wax, 68
　see also Otitis
Echymosis, 1
Electrolytes, 29
Emphysema surgical, 80
Empyema thoracis, 83
Embolus, 36
　Mesenteric, 118
　Pulmonary, 36
Endarterectomy, 35
Epididymitis, 205
Epilepsy, 147

Epiphisis slipped, 173
Epithelioma, 46
Ergot poisoning, 41
Ethanolamine, 43
Exophthalmos, 59

Faecal impaction, 119
Fissure-in-ano, 129
Fistula, 4
　in diverticulitis, 121
　in regional enteritis, 112
　Tracheo-oesophageal, 87
Fistula-in-ano, 128
Flail chest, 79
Fluid balance, 29
Fluid intravenous, 30
Fractures, 163
　Complications, 164
　General treatment, 165
　Mal-union, 164
　Types, 163
　of carpals, 167
　of clavicle, 166
　of facial, 165
　of femur, 167
　of forearm bones, 166, 167
　of humerus, 166
　of mandible, 166
　of metacarpals, 167
　of metatarsals, 170
　of nasal, 165
　of pelvis, 167
　of phalanges, 167, 170
　of rib, 79
　of skull, 143
　of spine, 152
　of tarsal, 170
　of tibia, 169
　of wrist, 167
　of zygoma, 166
Fracture-dislocation, 174
Frozen section, 76
Furuncle, 45

Gall bladder, 138
　Carcinoma, 141
　Cholecystitis, 139
Gall stones, 139
Ganglion, 177
Gangrene, 40
Gas gangrene, 13
Gastroscopy, 104
Glands, Tumours of, 17, 18
　(See also under gland or organ)
Glioma, 148
Glossitis, 53
Gigantism, 150
Goitre, 59
Grafts, Arterial, 39
　Skin, 48
　Types, 50
Granulation tissue, 3

Haemangioma, 17
Haematemesis, 108

Haematocele, 206
Haematoma, 1
  Subungal haematoma, 179
Haemorrhage, 34
  Intracrainial, 145
Haemorrhoids, 125
  Acute thrombosed, 126
Haemothorax, 81
Hallux valgus, 173
Hashimotos disease, 60
Heart, 84
  Acquired disease, 86
  Congenital disease, 84
Heartburn, 89
Heart lung machine, 86
Hellers operation, 89
Hepatoma, 133
Hernia, 98
  Epigastric, 101
  Femoral, 99
  Hiatus, 89
  Incisional, 101
  Inguinal, 98
  Parumbilical, 101
  Umbilical, 100
  Strangulated, 98
Herpes simples, 53
Herpid, 53
Hirschsprungs disease (See Colon)
Hydrocele, 206
Hydrocephalus, 149
Hydronephrosis, 184
Hyperhidrosis, 157
Hyperparathyroidism, 61
Hypoparathyroidism, 61
Hypospadias, 202

Infection, 9
  of hand and finger, 178
  of tendons, 177
  Body responses to, 9
  General complications of, 11
  Local complications of, 10
Ileostomy, For ulcerative colitis, 122
  For urinary diversion, 196
Infertility, 207
Inflammation, 9
Insulinoma, 136
Interverterbral disc, 154
  Prolapse of, 154
Intestines, 111
Intestinal obstruction, 114
Intussusception, 116
Isotope scan, Brain, 143
  Kidney, 182
  Liver, 139
  Whole body, 76

Joints, 171

Keloid, 3
Knee, torn cartilage of, 173
Kidney, 181
  Calculi, 186
  Carcinoma, 188

Kidney—contd.
  Cysts, 183
  Investigations, 182
  Nephroblastoma, 187
  Perinephric abscess, 186
  Polycystic disease, 183
  Pyelonephritis, 185
  Pyonephrosis, 185
  Rupture, 182
  Transplant, 189
Kopliks spots, 52
Kuntscher nail, 169

Labyrinthitis, 69
Laryngitis, 65
Larynx, 65
  Paralysis of, 66
  Tumours of, 65
Leucoplakia, 54
Leukaemia, 18
Lip, 51
  Cleft (hare), 51
  Infection, 53–54
  Malignant, 54
Lipoma, 17
Liver, 131
  Carcinoma, 133
  Cirrhosis, 132
  Hepatoma, 133
  Rupture, 132
  Scan, 139
Lockjaw, 12
Lung, 77
  Abscess, 83
  Embolism of, 36
  Tumours, 83
Lymphadenitis, 11, 15
  Mesenteric, 114
Lymphadenoma, 16
Lymphangiogram, 16
Lymphangitis, 11
Lymphoma, 16

Mastitis, 73
  Acute, 73
  Chronic, 74
Mastoiditis, 69
Melaena
  from peptic ulceration, 108
  from diverticulitis, 120
Melanoma malignant, 46
Menieres syndrome, 69
Meninges, 142
Meningioma, 148
Meningocele, 151
Meningomyelocele, 152
Mitral stenosis, 86
Mouth, 51
  Carcinoma, 52
  Inflammation (stomatitis), 52
  Ulcer, 52
Muscle rupture, 176
Myoma, 17

Nephroblastoma, 187

Neuroblastoma, 190
Nerve
　Injury, 157
　Peripheral, 156
　Sympathetic, 157
Neuroma, Auditory nerve, 148
Nose, 70
　Rhinitis, 70
　Polyps, 70
　Septal deviation, 70
　Tumours, 71
Noxyflex, 95

Oesophagitis, 89
Oesophagus, 87
　Achalasia, 88
　Atresia, 87
　Carcinoma, 90
　Investigations, 87
　Plummer-Vinson syndrome, 88
　Varices, 132
　Ulceration, 89
Onychogryphosis, 179
Orchitis, 205
Osteogenisis imperfecta, 161
Osteitis deformans, 160
Osteoarthritis, 172
Osteoclastoma, 161
Osteogenic sarcoma, 162
Osteoma, 161
Osteomalacia, 160
Osteomyelitis, Acute, 158
　Chronic, 159
Otits, Externa, 168
　Media, 169
　Secretory, 168

Palate, 51
　Cleft, 51
Pagets disease, 160
Pancreas, 135
　Adenoma, 136
　Carcinoma, 137
　Pseudo cyst, 136
Pancreatitis
　Acute, 135
　Relapsing, 136
Papilloma, 17
　(See also under organs)
Paralytic ileus, 96
Parathormone, 61
Parathyroid glands, 61
Paraphimosis, 203
Paronychia, 178
Parotid, 54
　Calculi, 55
　Tumours, 56
Parotitis, 55
Penis, 197
　Carcinoma, 203
　Warts, 203
Pentogastrin test, 104
Peptic ulcer, 104
　Acute, 104
　Chronic, 105

Perforation of, 107
Peritoneum, 93
Peritonitis
　Acute, 93
　Chronic, 96
Perthes disease, 173
Pharynx, 62
　Pouch, 64
　Tumours, 64
Pharyngitis, 63
Pituitary gland, 149
　Tumours, 150
Plasma, 32
　Substitutes, 33
Pleural effusion, 82
Plummer-Vinson syndrome, 88
Pneumothorax, 80
Polyps, of the bowel, 123
　Nasal, 70
Porta-caval shunt, 132
Potts fracture, 169
Pressure sore, 7
Proctitis, 130
Prolapse rectal, 127
Prostate, 197
　Benign hypertrophy, 198
　Carcinoma, 200
Prostatitis, Acute, 197
　Chronic, 198
Proud flesh, 3
Pruritus ani, 129
Pulmonary embolism, 36
Pulp infection, 179
Pyaemia, 11
Pyelonephritis, 185
Pyloric stenosis, Acquired, 108
　Congenital, 110
Pyonephrosis, 185

Rammstedt's operation, 110
Raynaud's disease, 41
Rectum, Adenoma of, 123
　Prolapse of, 127
　Carcinoma of, 125
　Ulcerative colitis of, 122
Regional enteritis, 111
Respiration, 78
　Paradoxical, 79
　Positive pressure, 79
Reticuloses, 16
Rhinitis, 70
Risus sardonicus, 13
Rodent ulcer, 46

Salazopyrin, 112
Salivary glands, 54
　Calculi of, 55
　Tumours of, 56
Scalp lacerations, 143
Scoliosis, 155
Sengstaken tube, 132
Septicaemia, 11
Sequestrum, 159
Shock, 25
　Causes of, 26

Shock—*contd.*
   Types of, 26
   Treatment of, 27
Sinus, 4
   Nasal, 71
   Pilonidal, 4
Sinusitis, 71
Skip lesions, 111
Skin, 45
   Flaps, 49
   Grafts, 48
   Infections of, 45
   Tumours of 17–18, 46
Spina bifida, 151
Spinal cord, 151
   Injury of, 153
   Tumours of, 155
Spleen, 133
Sprain, 174
Staphyloccus aureus, 12
Steatorrhora, 109
Stomach, 102
   Gastric ulcer, 106
   Hour glass, 109
   Carcinoma of, 109
Stomatitis, 52
Streptococcus pyogenes, 12
Streptokinase, 35
Sublingual gland, 55
Submandibular gland, 55
   Calculi of, 55
   Tumours of, 56

Talipes equino varus, 173
Tendon
   Achilles rupture, 176
   Division of, 177
   Quadriceps rupture, 176
Tenosynovitis
   Acute, 177
   Suppurative, 177
Tennis elbow, 176
Teratoma, 207
Testes, 204
   Inflammation of, 205
   Torsion of, 205
   Tumours of, 207
   Undescended, 204
Tetanus, 12
   Treatment of, 13
   Prevention of, 13
Tetany, 61
Thomas splint, 169
Thorax, 77
Thrombosis, 34
   Arterial, 34
   Mesenteric, 119
   Venous, 35

Thrombophlebitis, 35
Thrombus, 34
Thyroid gland, 58
   Adenoma of, 60
   Cyst of, 60
   Tumours of, 60
Thyrotoxicosis, 59
Thyroxin, 58
Toe nail, Ingrowing, 179
Tongue, 53
   Inflammation of, 53
   Tie, 53
   Ulcers of, 53
Tonsil, 62
   Hypertrophy of, 64
   Tonsillitis, 63
Transplant, Renal, 189
Tracheostomy, 66
Trigger finger, 177
Truss, 99
Tuberculosis, 14
   Treatment of, 14
   Bone, 159
Tumours, 17

Ulcers, 6–8
   Aphthous, 52
   Gastric, 106
   Malignant, 8
   Oesophageal, 89
   Peptic, 104
   Rodent, 46
   Stomal, 109
   Tuberculous, 8
   Varicose, 43
Ulcerative colitis (*See* Colon)
Urea, 30
Ureter, 181
   Calculi, 187
Urethra, 197
   Rupture, 201
   Stricture, 202
Urine retention, 200
Urinary diversions, 195

Varicocele, 206
Varicose veins, 42
   Eczema, 44
   Ulcer, 43
Vasectomy, 207
Ventriculography, 143
Volvulus, 117

Wounds, 1
Warts, Penile, 203
   Plantar, 180

Zollinger-Ellison syndrome, 136